T0288280

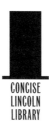

CONCISE
LINCOLN
LIBRARY

—

EDITED BY RICHARD W. ETULAIN,

SARA VAUGHN GABBARD, AND

SYLVIA FRANK RODRIGUE

GLENNA R. SCHROEDER-LEIN

Lincoln and Medicine

Southern Illinois University Press
Carbondale and Edwardsville

15 14 13 12   4 3 2 1

The Concise Lincoln Library has been made possible
in part through a generous donation by the Leland E.
and LaRita R. Boren Trust.

Library of Congress Cataloging-in-Publication Data
Schroeder-Lein, Glenna R., 1951–
Lincoln and medicine / Glenna R. Schroeder-Lein.
    p. cm. — (Concise Lincoln library)
Includes bibliographical references and index.
ISBN 978-0-8093-3194-9 (cloth : alk. paper)
ISBN 0-8093-3194-2 (cloth : alk. paper)
ISBN 978-0-8093-3195-6 (ebook)
ISBN 0-8093-3195-0 (ebook)
1. Lincoln, Abraham, 1809–1865—Health. 2. Lincoln,
Abraham, 1809–1865—Family—Health. I. Title.
E457.2.S375 2012
973.7092—dc23   2012003168

Printed on recycled paper. ♻
The paper used in this publication meets the mini-
mum requirements of American National Standard
for Information Sciences—Permanence of Paper for
Printed Library Materials, ANSI Z39.48-1992. ∞

For

Lonnie, again

also for
Mabel M. Lein
and in memory of
Martin O. Lein
(1920–2003)

CONTENTS

ILLUSTRATIONS

PREFACE

Did Abraham Lincoln have Marfan syndrome? Was Mary insane? What did Willie die from? Many questions have been asked about the health of Lincoln and his family members. While there have been a number of articles addressing various aspects of the health of the Lincolns, there has been no overview volume since *Lincoln and the Doctors: A Medical Narrative of the Life of Abraham Lincoln*, published by Milton H. Shutes in 1933, on the sixty-eighth anniversary of Lincoln's death. This book attempts to fill that gap.

Shutes focused not only on Lincoln's health but also on all the doctors Lincoln knew, even if they never treated him. This book does not include any of those doctors unless they are directly relevant to Lincoln's health. Shutes did not include source notes, often making it difficult to determine where he got his information. This volume does include source endnotes, using short titles, as well as a bibliography giving full title and publishing information.

In the roughly eighty years since Shutes published his book, Lincoln studies have taken many new turns, sometimes focusing on subjects unimaginable in the 1930s. This book attempts to take those new perspectives into account. Chapter 1 covers the young Lincoln, while chapter 2 focuses on the medical issues of Lincoln and his family during the Springfield years. The family focus continues in chapter 3, which discusses the period of Lincoln's presidency. Chapter 4 addresses many questions raised in the past several decades about whether Lincoln had such conditions as Marfan syndrome, ataxia, MEN2B, or mercury poisoning or had a homosexual orientation. Chapter 5

studies Lincoln's interaction with wartime medical issues, both personally and as commander in chief. Chapter 6 analyzes Lincoln's assassination, and chapter 7 briefly traces the postwar medical history of the
remaining members of the Lincoln family—Tad, Mary, and Robert.

Because this book is sharply focused on the subject of Lincoln and
medicine, readers desiring more biographical detail may consult several excellent single-volume studies such as David Herbert Donald's
Lincoln or Ronald C. White's *A. Lincoln: A Biography*. People who
would like some additional background in period medicine may find
useful the author's *The Encyclopedia of Civil War Medicine*, the classic
studies *Doctors in Blue* by George Worthington Adams and *Doctors
in Gray* by H. H. Cunningham, or Alfred Jay Bollet's more recent
Civil War Medicine: Challenges and Triumphs.

It is a privilege to thank those who have assisted and encouraged me
in this study. When Sylvia Frank Rodrigue mentioned the idea of the
Concise Lincoln Library and casually asked if I might be interested
in doing a volume, maybe Lincoln and medicine, I considered the
idea sort of a joke. Then I looked a little further and realized there
actually would be enough information. And here it is. Sylvia has
faithfully checked on my progress and provided great encouragement
throughout the process.

Colleagues at the Abraham Lincoln Presidential Library in Springfield, Illinois, have proved most helpful: Mary Ann Pohl and Jennifer
Ericson pulled items from the Lincoln Collection; Bob Cavanagh
procured books and articles through interlibrary loan; James Corne-
lius answered some questions and loaned me a DVD; Gwen Podeschi
and Dennis Suttles aided in various ways; and Cheryl Schnirring,
Cheryl Pence, and Kathryn Harris provided support as necessary. I
could not have done it without you.

Daniel Stowell, David Gerleman, and Sean Scott of the Papers of
Abraham Lincoln, and John Lupton, formerly of that project, helped
me to get copies of several useful documents. Jason Emerson supplied
some information about Robert Todd Lincoln. Members of several
Bible studies were a crucial support. Many thanks to Kathy, Rich,
Joyce, Linda, Vince, Lin, Glen, Marilyn, Tom, Doris, Irene, John,

Shonté, Dan, Chris, Jason, and Agnes. My husband's colleagues at WLUJ Christian radio allowed me to spend two very productive days writing in their basement room. Cynthia Needham provided exceptional encouragement at a number of Panera brunches.

Special thanks to Tom Schwartz, Jack Navins, and Michael Hiranuma for reading and commenting on the entire manuscript. Tom's expertise, helpful materials, and periodic discussions on Lincoln questions eased some of the challenges of writing a Lincoln book. Jack supplied some crucial material on DNA and served as my medical reader. Michael demonstrated his longtime friendship by reading a second book for me and catching some important details. I cannot thank all of you enough!

My husband, Lonnie Lein, was surprised that I would want to take on another book, especially after the medical encyclopedia. He thinks I should dedicate this volume to him for putting up with me through writing four books. He is right, of course, so I have done as he wished. This book is also dedicated to Mabel M. Lein and to the memory of Martin O. Lein. I could not have asked for better in-laws.

LINCOLN AND MEDICINE

YOUNG LINCOLN, 1809–42

As most people know, Abraham Lincoln was born near Hodgenville, Kentucky, on February 12, 1809, the second child of Thomas and Nancy Hanks Lincoln. Abraham had an older sister, Sarah, and a younger brother, Thomas, who died in infancy. The family moved to a farm on Knob Creek in 1811 but soon left Kentucky entirely, moving to Indiana in late 1816. Abraham's mother died on October 5, 1818, of milk sickness, a disease spread through the milk of cows that have eaten a poisonous plant. Thomas Lincoln remarried just over a year later. The extended family located in Illinois in 1830. The following year, Abraham moved away from home, ending up in the town of New Salem.

Little information beyond the basics survives about Abraham Lincoln's childhood and youth. The majority of it is in reminiscences collected from friends and acquaintances by his former law partner William H. Herndon after Lincoln's death. Only a tiny fraction of that information pertains to incidents of Lincoln's health.

Lincoln apparently had a relatively healthy childhood, as testified by his stepmother, Sarah Bush Johnston Lincoln. She claimed he "never was sick" and was "more fleshy" when the family lived in Indiana than after they moved to Illinois. Lincoln did experience several accidents, however. When the family still resided in Kentucky, Lincoln and a young friend, Austin Gollaher, were trying to cross Knob Creek on a log. Lincoln fell into five or six feet of water and probably would have drowned if Gollaher had not rescued him.[1]

A further traumatic incident occurred in Indiana when Lincoln was nine, one that Lincoln even mentioned himself. He had taken grain to Noah Gordon's mill. To speed up the horse at the grindstone, Lincoln shouted and hit the animal with a whip. The horse kicked Lincoln in the head, knocking him out, or as Lincoln phrased it, he was "apparently killed for a time." When he came to, Lincoln finished the sentence he had started before he was kicked, an action that several people have suggested was indicative of petit mal epileptic seizures that Lincoln then supposedly experienced for the rest of his life.[2] Although there is little evidence for further seizure episodes, Lincoln may have suffered other permanent injuries. He possibly had nerve damage, causing his eyelid to droop and the corner of his mouth to curl on one side. The head injury may also have contributed to his later headaches. Some have suggested that Lincoln's eye misalignment and occasional jerking of the left eye were results of being kicked by the horse. Others have pointed out that Lincoln's son Robert and several other relatives had various eye problems, so the condition was probably hereditary, perhaps a form of crossed eyes.[3]

As a young man of nineteen, Lincoln, with Allen Gentry, started from Indiana and took a flatboat of cargo down the Mississippi River to New Orleans. "[O]ne night they were attacked by seven negroes with intent to kill and rob them. They were hurt some in the melee, but succeeded in driving the negroes from the boat" and quickly pushed away from shore, Lincoln reported in his 1860 autobiography. Apparently the injuries were not severe. Given Lincoln's avid participation in wrestling and other physical sports, it would be surprising if he did not experience some minor injuries while engaging in those activities as well, but nothing has been recorded about them. Lincoln and his family all seem to have had malaria in the fall of 1830, soon after they moved to the Decatur, Illinois, area. This illness apparently helped motivate them to move again soon after. Lincoln may also have had malaria during the summer of 1835 when he was living in New Salem.[4]

One of Lincoln's health issues, which was a topic of discussion during his lifetime and remains a subject of considerable interest, was his mental state, especially the matter of his depressions and melancholy.

Lincoln had two major incidents of depression that lasted more than a week. The first occurred during the late summer of 1835. A friend of his, Ann Rutledge, had died on August 25, probably of typhoid fever. The exact nature of Lincoln's relationship to Ann has been a source of contention and discussion since November 16, 1866, when William H. Herndon proclaimed in a lecture that Ann had been Lincoln's one true love and Lincoln had never loved his wife, Mary.[5] Some of Herndon's New Salem informants had never known of any romantic involvement between Lincoln and Ann. Others claimed the two had been engaged. In either case, Lincoln does seem to have taken her death unusually hard and been very depressed. Elizabeth Abell, with whose family Lincoln was living at the time, later reported to Herndon that during one storm Lincoln remarked that "he could not bare the idea of its raining on her Grave." Although some others from the community told Herndon that Lincoln had been "crazy" and they were afraid he would commit suicide, Abell denied the charge, indicating that Lincoln simply "was very disponding a long time."[6]

Joshua Shenk, who has written a substantial volume on Lincoln's struggle with depression, has suggested that just because Lincoln's depressive episode began soon after Ann Rutledge's death does not mean that her death caused the depression. Several of Herndon's informants noted that Lincoln's severe upset was triggered by bad weather. Others mentioned that Lincoln had been studying law very intensely and eating poorly. The depression could well have been caused by a combination of stresses.[7] If Milton H. Shutes was correct that Lincoln had malaria during the summer of 1835, physical illness could also have been a factor in Lincoln's depression. Unfortunately, Shutes did not indicate his sources in his 1933 study, and none of Herndon's informants seem to mention chills and fever, so the possibility cannot be substantiated at present.[8]

Lincoln suffered his second major depression in Springfield, Illinois, where he had moved to practice law in 1837. This depression began in late December 1840 or early January 1841. On January 23, Lincoln forced himself to write to his law partner John T. Stuart, lamenting, "I am now the most miserable man living. If what I feel were equally distributed to the whole human family, there would not be one cheerful face on the earth. Whether I shall ever be better I cannot tell; I awfully forbode I shall not. To remain as I am is impossible; I must die or be better, it appears to me."[9]

Traditionally, because of a later reference to the "fatal first of Jany." in a letter from Lincoln to his good friend Joshua Speed, most people have assumed that Lincoln and his eventual wife, Mary Todd, broke their engagement on January 1, 1841, and that this caused Lincoln's depression. A few have even suggested that he left her standing at the altar on that date. In reality, no one knows when Lincoln and Mary broke up, or why. Various explanations include opposition to the match from Mary's Springfield relatives; Mary's flirtation with Stephen A. Douglas or other men; Lincoln's realization that he did not love Mary but was interested in Matilda Edwards, a young visitor in town who also interested Joshua Speed; and Lincoln's discovery that Mary was emotionally unstable.

Yet it is entirely possible that Lincoln and Mary's breakup was only a part of the problem. Lincoln had barely been reelected to the state legislature for a fourth term in August 1840. There he continued to be a leading advocate of "internal improvements," the state funding of canals, railroads, and other developments that, due to the panic beginning in 1837, had caused Illinois serious state debt. Several incidents in the legislature in December 1840 were embarrassing to Lincoln and suggested that his political career might soon be ending. Lincoln had campaigned vigorously in Illinois in the fall for William Henry Harrison, probably exhausting himself, only to see Harrison lose Illinois even though he won the presidency. In addition, the weather was again dismal in December 1840 and January 1841.

Possibly worst of all, Joshua Speed was selling his portion of his store, effective January 1, 1841, and was planning to move back to Kentucky. Since Speed and Lincoln had shared living quarters for four years, ever since Lincoln had moved to Springfield, and were very close friends, this was certainly a blow for Lincoln emotionally and relationally.[10]

Whatever the cause of Lincoln's distress, the resulting episode was quite dramatic. He had some kind of illness or breakdown. Friends, including Speed, said Lincoln went crazy and they had to keep razors and knives away from him. During January 1841, Lincoln missed about a week of sessions of the state legislature, which he normally would have attended faithfully. Diagnosed with "hypochondriasis" (thinking a condition is serious when it is not), Lincoln evidently spent the week in bed being treated by Dr. Anson G. Henry, his faithful political and personal friend. No one knows what the treatments were, but a number of historians have speculated that because Henry was a follower of Dr. Benjamin Rush of Philadelphia, the remedies could have included "heroic" bleeding, purging, blistering, and other unpleasant ministrations. What is known is that when Lincoln emerged from the treatment, he was not cured and was very weak. Although Lincoln was doing much better in February, he was still recovering in July and August 1841 when he went to Kentucky to visit Joshua Speed and his family.[11]

Most scholars agree that Lincoln had only the two major depressions discussed, although a few think that even those episodes do not qualify as major depressions. However, many people throughout Lincoln's life remarked on his evident and frequent sadness, as Lincoln himself did.[12]

A number of people have endeavored to determine the cause of Lincoln's sadness or melancholy. Lincoln's legal colleagues John T. Stuart and Leonard Swett blamed his melancholy on digestive problems, including poor bile secretion from the liver that resulted in chronic constipation. Treatment of this condition with large doses of calomel (a mercurial preparation) has also been indicated as a factor. Malaria, bad teeth, and bad feet have been suggested as causes, as well as the effects of pioneer hardships and the early deaths of his mother and sister. In the 1920s and 1930s, it was popular to suggest that Lincoln had some sort of thyroid problem that contributed to his melancholy. Some have blamed Lincoln's temperament and suggested that melancholy was hereditary, suffered by other relatives as well. Others have cited his marriage to Mary Todd as a cause of depression, but Lincoln clearly suffered from depression or melancholy long before his marriage, as well as during it.[13]

A question often discussed recently is whether Lincoln had chronic depression or just a melancholy temperament. Author John G. Sotos's contention that Lincoln was not melancholy at all but looked that way when he was "thinking" because he had low facial muscle tone may be ignored as special pleading to prove Lincoln had another disease, MEN2B.[14]

Joshua Shenk, author of the book *Lincoln's Melancholy*, is the chief advocate of the view that Lincoln suffered chronic depression (not bipolar or manic depression), basing his conclusion on the numerous accounts of Lincoln's bouts of sadness or melancholy as well as on much recent psychological research. After the 1841 depression episode, Lincoln was much more self-controlled, not giving way to anguish as he had done twice previously. Based on the same sources that Shenk uses, those who argue that Lincoln had a melancholy temperament do not see him as any less depressed than Shenk does. Instead, melancholy was an aspect of his personality, not an illness responsive to stimuli from particular situations. As summarized by historian Doris Kearns Goodwin, Lincoln's melancholy did not immobilize him but enabled him to function, even as president, in a well-balanced way.[15]

No matter which side a person might take, and in many respects the viewpoints differ only in degree, nearly everyone agrees that Lincoln dealt well with his emotional struggles. His frequent use of funny stories in various situations, as well as his love of poetry and Shakespeare, was a type of therapy for him, as he even mentioned himself. It would seem that in Lincoln's case, as in many others, a melancholy temperament could actually aid a person in the development of their abilities.[16]

Lincoln, of course, suffered some of the miscellaneous ills that everyone suffers. In December 1838, he was sick while in Vandalia, Illinois, attending the state legislature. Apparently the ailment lingered on, and Lincoln became somewhat depressed. During the summer of 1841, while Lincoln was in Kentucky visiting the Speeds, he had a painful problem with one of his teeth. Unable to get it pulled there, he had it done in Springfield in September. Unfortunately, a part of the jawbone came out with the tooth, leaving Lincoln in too much pain to talk or eat for more than a week. At some point, Lincoln also had an accident with an ax, leaving a scar on his left forefinger.[17]

One further medical issue relates to the period before Lincoln's marriage. Did Lincoln have syphilis? In the nineteenth century, syphilis was not curable. Because the disease can progress to debilitating and even fatal stages, it is not surprising that many feared it. There was also some confusion about how it was transmitted. A number of people worried needlessly because they feared infection from passing, nonsexual contact.[18]

The whole question arises because of a single statement by William H. Herndon to his friend and collaborator Jesse W. Weik. Herndon claimed that Lincoln told him that he had gotten syphilis sometime in 1835 or 1836 when he "went to Beardstown and during a devilish passion had Connection with a girl and Caught the disease." There also have been suggestions that Joshua Speed visited prostitutes and may have referred Lincoln to one of them on occasion. Over time, most historians have been dubious, but more recently some have been more inclined to believe Herndon. Although John Sotos, a medical doctor, claimed that "there is an astonishing Lincoln syphilophobia among his admirers," historians have several good arguments to back their doubts that Lincoln actually had syphilis.[19]

Historians have had a love-hate relationship with Herndon. Although they have to rely on the material he collected in order to write their accounts of Lincoln's early life, many do not fully trust Herndon and his information. The syphilis story would be a case in point. Herndon wrote about it to Weik more than fifty years after it allegedly happened and more than twenty years after Lincoln's death. Lincoln hardly ever made confessions to anyone, including Herndon (much to Herndon's chagrin), and he never told Joshua Speed or anyone else this story. Some have suggested that Lincoln wrote to the noted physician Daniel Drake in Cincinnati to ask for a treatment for syphilis, while others believe Lincoln was writing for a treatment for depression. Speed knew Lincoln wrote the letter to Drake but did not know the subject. In any case, Drake refused to treat Lincoln without a personal examination, and Lincoln's letter to Drake has never turned up.[20] Doctors who have assessed the question have found no evidence that Lincoln ever contracted syphilis. He displayed none of the obvious symptoms and would have had about thirty years to do so.[21]

Despite some bouts of depression, malaria, and occasional common illnesses, as well as a few injuries, Lincoln was evidently in generally good physical health as he began the next phase of his life. As Lincoln phrased it, it was a "matter of profound wonder"—he got married.[22]

THE LINCOLN FAMILY, 1843–60

When Abraham Lincoln married Mary Todd on November 4, 1842, he took on new responsibilities for family members, as do most married men. In Lincoln's case, his relationship with his wife has been studied extensively, if not excessively, from their first meeting to their last words to each other on April 14, 1865. It is important to reiterate that the details of that relationship are important to the topic of this chapter only as they relate to the health of the family members.

Mary Ann Todd was born December 13, 1818, in Lexington, Kentucky, the fourth child of Robert Smith and Eliza Parker Todd. Mary's mother died when Mary was six. After her father remarried less than two years later, neither Mary nor her five full siblings ever got along well with their stepmother, Elizabeth (Betsey) Humphreys, who produced nine additional children.[1] Little seems to be known about Mary's physical health as a child. More attention has been paid to her emotional and mental conditions in light of her later instability. The description by Mary's cousin Margaret Stuart Woodrow, one of Mary's best friends as a child, has been quoted often: "She was very highly strung, nervous, impulsive, excitable, having an emotional temperament much like an April day, sunning all over with laughter one moment, the next crying as though her heart would break." Mary's mood swings, equally evident in adulthood, have led some to suggest that she was bipolar (manic-depressive).[2] Several historians have noted that Mary was not properly disciplined as a

child, a situation also true for many of her siblings. She did not develop self-control but became self-centered and demanding. By the
time she went to live with her oldest sister, Elizabeth Edwards, in
Springfield, Illinois, in 1839, Mary had also begun to experience the
severe headaches or migraines from which she suffered for the rest
of her life. She may also have learned how useful illness could be in
getting attention and her own way.[3]

In addition to the common transitions involved in adjusting to
being married, Mary faced two extra challenges. She moved from
the Edwards home, with servants and society events, to the Globe
Tavern, a boardinghouse. Mary immediately became pregnant as
well. The shift from society belle to pregnant wife of a rising but still
lower-income lawyer was not an easy adjustment for Mary.[4]

The couple's first son, Robert Todd Lincoln, called Bob by the
family, was born August 1, 1843. Robert evidently took after his
mother's side of the family physically. His father described him when
three years old as "'short and low,' and I expect always will be." At
that age he talked "plainly," was "quite smart enough," and got into
mischief. At some point, the young Bob "ate poisonous lime from the
Lincoln privy." Although this was certainly nasty and very upsetting
to Mary, it apparently did the boy no lasting damage.[5]

Perhaps one of the scariest events of Robert's childhood for the
Lincoln family occurred when Robert was bitten by his dog. Apparently
the Lincolns feared that the dog had hydrophobia (rabies), for which
no effective preventative or treatment then existed. However, Abraham
Lincoln did what any loving parent would do to provide the best medical care available. He took Robert all the way to Terre Haute, Indiana,
to be treated with a "mad stone." These rare stones were supposed to
draw out the poison. Needless to say, the dog was not really rabid.
However, the incident does show the Lincolns as caring parents, as
well as the limits of effective treatment at the time.[6]

Robert's most obvious medical issue during his childhood was
a crossed eye, a situation that led to severe teasing by his school-
mates, who taunted him with the name "Cockeye." Studies of Robert
and the Lincoln family during his childhood mention several different treatments for this apparently hereditary problem. He may have

strengthened the eye by the use of a patch or by peering through a keyhole. It is also possible that he had surgery on the affected eye muscles. Unfortunately, none of the historians who mention these treatments indicate their original sources, so it is impossible to determine for sure what may have been done to Robert's eye. Evidently the procedures were not fully successful, however, as photos later in life show a slight turning in of the left eye. Reportedly, Robert eventually lost the sight in that eye as well. One author tried to suggest that Robert's eye problem was a sign of Marfan syndrome, a connective tissue disorder also attributed to Abraham Lincoln, but had to admit that this was very unlikely since Robert lived to be almost eighty-three and most untreated Marfan sufferers die early.[7]

Edward Baker Lincoln, called Eddie (or Eddy), joined the family on March 10, 1846. Named for one of Lincoln's political friends, Eddie apparently took after the Lincoln side of the family. His father reported to Joshua Speed that Eddie was "rather of a longer order" than Robert. Eddie had several illnesses in 1848, in May and in the fall, but their nature is not known. Eddie became sick again in mid-December 1849 and was ill for fifty-two days before he died at six o'clock on the morning of February 1, 1850. The funeral was held at the Lincoln home the following morning, and Eddie was buried in Hutchinson's cemetery.[8]

Two main causes of death have been proposed for Eddie. The first is diphtheria. Researcher Milton Shutes, in an article about the mortality of the Lincoln boys, made a lengthy argument for the disease, based initially on an erroneous transcription of Lincoln's letter that said Eddie was sick for *fifteen* days. Although diphtheria made more sense as a cause of death after the shorter illness, Shutes continued to explain why diphtheria could also cause death after fifty-two days. He did admit that there was no direct evidence for the disease, however. Several other scholars accepted diphtheria as the probable cause of Eddie's death.[9]

The second suggested fatal disease comes from the 1850 mortality schedule, a part of the census that listed the cause of death for those who died during the census year. As discovered by indefatigable researcher Wayne Temple, the mortality schedule showed that Eddie had died from "consumption," now more commonly called tuberculosis. This contemporary diagnosis makes more sense in light of the fifty-two-day illness and the suggestions that Eddie was generally a sickly child. Unfortunately, Temple at that time (1966) espoused the idea that Eddie "must have suffered also from the Marfan Syndrome," an idea for which there is no evidence but only speculation. Tuberculosis is now more commonly accepted as the cause of Eddie's death.[10]

The Lincoln family grieved the loss of Eddie. As Lincoln wrote to his stepbrother, "We miss him very much." Part of the grieving process apparently included either or both parents writing a memorial poem, "Little Eddie," which was published in the *Illinois Journal* on February 7, 1850. Eddie's death was especially difficult for Mary as it closely followed the deaths of her father in a cholera epidemic during the summer of 1849 and of her grandmother Parker during Eddie's illness. Some historians have suggested that this string of losses changed Mary's personality for the worse.[11]

Mary was soon pregnant again, and William Wallace Lincoln, named for the physician husband of Mary's sister Frances, was born December 21, 1850. Mary may have recovered somewhat slowly from Willie's birth; on January 12, 1851, Lincoln used the fact that she was "sick-abed" with "a case of baby-sickness" as one of the reasons why he could not go to visit his dying father. Mary evidently nursed Willie until he was at least seventeen months old.[12]

Willie no doubt had a variety of illnesses as a young child. The most serious, and the one about which something is known, was his bout with scarlet fever during June and July 1860. Because Lincoln was then the Republican presidential candidate, Willie's illness was even mentioned in the *Chicago Press and Tribune*, although the journalists erred in listing him as six years old. The paper also reported that the child was "lying ill at the point of death," and because "the parent is superior to the politician; Mr. Lincoln has not been seen outside of his house." Lincoln clarified this situation in a letter to his physician friend Anson G. Henry on July 4, 1860: Willie "has just had a hard and tedious spell of scarlet fever; and he is not yet beyond all danger. I have a head-ache, and a sore throat upon me now, inducing me to suspect that I have an inferior type of the same thing." Several historians have suggested that this illness probably weakened Willie's constitution, making him susceptible to further illness.[13]

The youngest Lincoln son, Thomas, was named after Lincoln's father but was always called Tad, short for Tadpole. Born on April 4, 1853, Tad reportedly had a rather large head and scrawny body, leading to his nickname. Unfortunately for Mary, the large head caused her some injury during childbirth, possibly to her urethra, from which she never fully recovered. The injury may also account for the fact that the Lincolns had only four children.[14]

Tad was a wild, undisciplined child with mood swings that suggested a personality much like Mary's. He had a speech impediment that was very noticeable when the family lived in the White House. Perhaps born with a partially cleft lip and palate, Tad apparently had delayed language development and enunciation problems, possibly related to some dental issues. The speech and language pathologist who analyzed the recollections about Tad's language difficulties also suggested that the boy had some attention deficit hyperactivity disorder problems.[15]

In February 1859, Tad developed some sort of respiratory infection. Lincoln was attending to law business in Chicago, and on February 28 Mary attempted to send him a message by way of Ozias M. Hatch, Illinois secretary of state. She wrote to Hatch, "If you are going up to Chicago to day, & should meet Mr L—— there, will you say to him, that our *dear little Taddie*, is quite sick. The Dr thinks it may prove a *slight* attack of *lung* fever. I am feeling troubled & it would be a comfort to have him, *at home*. He passed a bad night, I do not like his symptoms, and will be glad, if he hurries home." It cannot now be determined how sick Tad really was, whether the illness had any permanent effect, or whether Lincoln cut short his business and came home. The letter does demonstrate Mary's great anxiety when any of the children were sick, which is not surprising after Eddie's death.[16]

While the Lincoln family undoubtedly experienced far more illnesses in the 1840s and 1850s than are indicated here, any knowledge of them depends on the survival of correspondence and other sources containing the proper information. For example, on August 31, 1851, Lincoln informed his stepbrother that "we are all well." But some unnamed member of the family was not well on January 12, 1854, preventing Lincoln from speaking at the Illinois State Colonization

Society annual meeting at Springfield. Lincoln himself was evidently "a little unwell when he left" for legal work in Chicago on or before March 2, 1857. When Lincoln was in Exeter, New Hampshire, in March 1860, he wrote to Mary after learning that "Willie and Taddy were very sick the Saturday night after I left." Having heard nothing further, he hoped they were well again.[17]

William Wallace, Mary's brother-in-law, was the family doctor much of the time the Lincolns lived in Springfield. If he was unavailable, his partner, Preston H. Bailhache, treated the Lincoln boys and collected the fees for medical services. Anson G. Henry treated Lincoln in 1841 and probably some other family members later. However, Henry was not always living in Springfield, having gone to Oregon in 1852, so he could not provide medical care. Amos W. French apparently cared for the Lincolns' dental needs in Springfield.[18]

There were several drugstores in Springfield to fill prescriptions and provide other medicines and remedies. Some of the ledgers from the Corneau and Diller store survive, including accounts for the Lincoln family. While it is possible to see what the Lincolns bought in 1855–60, it is not possible to determine who needed the remedy because individual names are not listed. One purchase that raised some later eyebrows was fifty cents' worth of "cocaine" on October 12, 1860. Harry Pratt, in his *Personal Finances of Abraham Lincoln*, assumed that this was a misspelling of cocaine, an interpretation followed by other historians. Cocaine was not a controlled substance in 1860, or for many years thereafter. However, journalist and historian Tara McClellan McAndrew discovered that cocaine was first prepared in Germany in 1860 and was not yet available elsewhere. Instead, she found that the Lincolns had purchased Burnett's Cocoaine, a hair tonic made from "cocoanut" oil and advertised in the *Illinois State Register*.[19]

Another medication of the period, commonly prescribed for a variety of ailments including the hypochondriasis and constipation attributed to Lincoln, was blue mass (a lump form) or blue pills, which combined various binding ingredients with calomel, a mercury preparation. Ward Hill Lamon, one of Lincoln's legal colleagues, told William Herndon that Lincoln always got a sick headache as a result of constipation and would take blue pills to relieve his discomfort.

Lincoln also took the pills for a few months around the time he went to Washington to become president, but he told John T. Stuart that he soon discontinued them because they made him cross.[20]

Based on these statements, physician Norbert Hirschhorn and several colleagues posited that Lincoln had low-level mercury poisoning, known as "micromercurialism." They speculated that in the 1850s, Lincoln exhibited "bizarre behavior and outbursts of rage, insomnia and forgetfulness," with hands "seen to tremble under stress," all symptoms of mercury poisoning. They believed that Lincoln's peculiar flat-footed walk might also be a symptom. All the other symptoms, except his walking style, supposedly diminished after Lincoln stopped taking the blue pills. Hirschhorn and his coworkers found an 1879 recipe for the pills, had some chemist friends make them up, and tested them. They found that the mercury content was 9,000 times what is currently considered an allowable amount.[21]

This was obviously strong medicine. Yet these figures do not necessarily mean anything for Lincoln since the recipe dated from fourteen years after Lincoln's death. Doctors and druggists manufactured their own pills; the medicine was not mass-produced and certainly varied. Furthermore, the evidence about Lincoln's alleged actions in the 1850s was not contemporary but collected by Herndon or even later historians. While it is certain that Lincoln took blue pills, no one knows when he began taking them, how often he took them, how strong they were, or when he stopped taking them. Hirschhorn counted the Lincolns' items in the Corneau and Diller record and found that of 245 purchases, only five were unspecified pills, and four were calomel. Nothing was noted as blue mass or blue pills for the Lincolns, although this medicine was listed for other customers. Hirschhorn and his coauthors speculated that Lincoln might have gotten them from the druggists "off the books," from Dr. Wallace, or from other drugstores on the legal circuit. Lincoln might in fact have done this. But it seems unlikely that he would have resorted to the clandestine measures Hirschhorn suggests. Regardless of the fact that Lincoln was running for public office, there would have been no reason to hide the purchase of blue pills, because they were so widely used for so many ailments. In all probability, Lincoln did not buy blue pills from Corneau and Diller because he did not take them consistently, only when necessary. While Lincoln at times suffered unpleasant side effects, such as cross moods, from the blue pills, it is unlikely that he took enough of them to experience full-fledged mercury poisoning, as proposed by Hirschhorn and his colleagues.[22]

Much has been said about Lincoln's medical difficulties, but it should be pointed out that he did several things that modern doctors suggest promote good health. According to his friend Ward Hill Lamon, Lincoln "loved apples better than all Else." Although Lamon claimed that Lincoln "took but little physical Exercise," that may depend on what a person considers to be exercise. Mary's sister Frances Wallace reported that Lincoln had a woodpile in the backyard where "he used to Saw wood for Exercise—he really loved to do it."[23]

As Lincoln aged, he, like many other people, became somewhat far-sighted. As a result, he bought his first pair of reading glasses at a store in Bloomington, Illinois, for 37½ cents in May 1856. He used low-grade lenses in several strengths for the rest of his life. Some doctors have suggested that some of these lenses were too strong and contributed to eyestrain and headaches on occasion.[24]

One other vision issue may be mentioned. Shortly after he was elected president, Lincoln lay down to rest and saw a double image of his face in a mirror. He moved around, and it disappeared. When he returned to his original position, he saw it again, but this was the only time it ever happened. Mary believed this was an omen that Lincoln would be elected twice but not live out his second term. Later commentators have been divided over whether Lincoln had an isolated episode of actual double vision or whether it was some sort of optical illusion.[25]

On May 18, 1860, delegates of the Republican Party, meeting in Chicago, selected Abraham Lincoln as their nominee for president. Lincoln's election to that office on November 6 provided him and his family with a new environment that included incredible stresses as well as exposure to more diseases than the Lincolns could ever have imagined.

THE LINCOLN FAMILY IN
WASHINGTON, DC, 1861–65

On February 11, 1861, a chilly, drizzly morning in Springfield, Illinois, Abraham Lincoln spoke poignant words of farewell to his friends and boarded the train for a lengthy trip to Washington, DC. In order to allow many people across the North to see their new president-elect, Lincoln's route was not the most direct and included brief stops at many small towns, as well as receptions and other festivities in the larger cities. Such a schedule was very tiring. Lincoln soon gave evidence of a severe cold and became so hoarse that he could barely be heard. He had to save his voice for the major cities.[1]

Once Lincoln had been inaugurated on March 4, the stresses related to the presidency that as early as December 1860 had made him "more pale and careworn than heretofore" only increased.[2] Two issues created the most concern. Patronage—filling politically appointed offices, from cabinet members to the lowly postmaster of a tiny village—consumed incredible amounts of a president's time in the days before civil service exams and appointments. Candidates came to call or sent their representatives, while copious amounts of mail arrived with letters of recommendation. In addition to these decisions, Lincoln had to determine what to do about the crisis caused by the secession of a number of Southern states, an unprecedented situation in the country's history. Lincoln found himself nearly overwhelmed. As Senator William P. Fessenden wrote home on March 17, "Our poor President is having a hard time of it. He came here tall, strong, and vigorous, but has worked himself almost to death. The good fellow thinks it is his duty to see to everything, and to do everything himself and consequently does many things foolishly." While foolishness may be a matter of opinion, Lincoln unquestionably was overworking himself. He had trouble sleeping. On March 30, Lincoln had a "sick headache" (probably a migraine) and fainted. He felt so poorly from the stress that he was unable to see any visitors on April 1.[3]

About this time, Mary took matters in hand and insisted that Lincoln have a daily carriage ride for rest and fresh air, which also gave the couple some much-needed time together. In addition, Mary tried to be sure Lincoln ate more regularly. He tended to start work as early as 5:00 A.M. without having had anything to eat. Mary sometimes invited company to breakfast so that Lincoln would have to attend. Lincoln's Illinois friend Orville H. Browning urged him to restrict his office hours for his own health. After the episode at the end of March, Lincoln did limit his office hours, seeing visitors only from 10:00 A.M. to 1:00 P.M.[4]

Lincoln was not alone in having some medical problems in March 1861. No sooner did the family get to Washington than Willie and Tad came down with measles. John Nicolay, one of Lincoln's private secretaries, reported that they were sick on March 20. Elizabeth Todd Grimsley, Mary's cousin who lived in the White House for the first six months of Lincoln's term, helped nurse the boys and reported that they had contracted measles from visiting the soldiers in the nearby army camps. This may be true, for measles were epidemic among new recruits throughout the war. However, the young men quartered in the capital about the time of the inauguration were mainly regular army or Washington militia and thus less likely to be rural recruits not previously exposed to measles. Although the newspapers reported the boys to be quite sick, Mary assured a correspondent that they had mild cases. The Lincoln family's young friend Elmer Ellsworth, a former law student of Lincoln's, caught measles as well, from the Lincoln boys, he believed. While the boys were sick, Lincoln would come in for a cup of tea and lunch and then lie on a couch reading to Willie and Tad from the Bible or some other book or quoting poetry. The boys also amused themselves with some illustrated Chinese books.[5]

As if two boys with measles were not bad enough, one evening within the first couple weeks after the inauguration, "every member of the family except the servants, was taken ill," Elizabeth Todd Grimsley reported. Doctors arrived and rumors spread that the family had been poisoned. "It proved to be only an over-indulgence in Potomac Shad, a new and tempting dish to western palates." From a modern perspective, it seems clear that the Lincolns suffered from some form of food poisoning, because they would not all have reacted digestively in the same way to food that was simply different. Possibly the fish had spoiled, been prepared with contaminated ingredients, or picked up some of the pollution from the Potomac River. In any case, the Lincolns quickly recovered.[6]

The family's first physician in Washington was Dr. John Richards, an Irish native who had immigrated to the United States in the 1830s and had been practicing medicine in Washington since 1852. His service to the Lincolns is generally not known because it was relatively short. Richards died January 19, 1862. Lincoln later endorsed Richards's widow's application for a copyist job.[7]

During the first summer of the war, Robert was ill as well. He telegraphed on July 17, 1861, from Harvard, where he was a student, letting his parents know that he had the mumps but was "not sick at all." He expected to be in Washington "in a few days" and was, in fact, there by August 3 when he attended festivities for Prince Napoleon of France.[8]

That same summer, Lincoln evidently had malaria. On August 31, Secretary of State William H. Seward's family visited Lincoln in his office. Seward's wife, Frances, noted in her diary that Lincoln "looks sick and is I fear threatened with intermitting fever—the room was awfully hot with gas and a wood fire." Probably Lincoln was in a chills phase of malaria.[9]

Also that summer, Mary, all three boys, and several other friends went to the beach at Long Branch, New Jersey, on vacation. They left Washington on August 14 and by the end of the month had gone on to Niagara Falls and New York City. Tad apparently had a bad cold while they were away. The family returned September 5, which was not late enough in the season for Mary to avoid malaria herself. She had "chills" in late September and early October 1861. Mary wrote her cousin Elizabeth Todd Grimsley on September 29 that "this is *my day of rest*, so I am sitting up—I am beginning to feel very weak." Mary evidently had one of the varieties of malaria where attacks of chills and fever did not occur every day. It reminded her of "the *early days*—when I used to have chills in Ill." She told Grimsley, "If they [the chills] cannot be broken in a few days, Mr Lincoln wants me to go North, & remain until cold weather." At that point the mosquitoes would die, eliminating the threat for new malaria cases in Washington. However, no one understood that it was the cold weather killing the mosquitoes that ended the malaria season; female anopheles mosquitoes were not discovered to be the spreaders of the disease until long after the Civil War. Mary was beginning to feel better by October 6, so she apparently did not go north for her health at that time.[10]

Although Mary Lincoln was not well enough to receive visitors on January 26, 1862, nothing else is known about the Lincoln family's health during the winter of 1861–62 until Willie became ill. Willie loved riding his new pony and evidently did so in bad weather. In late January or very early February, according to Elizabeth Keckly, Mary Lincoln's seamstress, confidant, and nurse, Willie caught "a severe cold, which deepened into fever. He was very sick." Mary sent for Keckly. Of course, the Lincolns also called their family physician, Dr. Robert K. Stone. Mary was particularly concerned because she had scheduled a large invitation-only party at the White House for February 5 and wondered if she should cancel it. Dr. Stone assured her that Willie was not in danger and she could hold the party. Unfortunately, Willie got much sicker the evening of the gathering. Keckly stayed with him during the event, but Mary left the festivities more than once to check on her son, who was feverish and having trouble breathing. Willie was even sicker the next day. Lincoln's secretary John Nicolay reported to his future wife, Therena Bates, that Lincoln spent most of the next few days with his sick son, whose condition fluctuated from somewhat better to critically ill. By February 10, Tad was sick as well. The Lincolns canceled receptions at the White House on February 8, 11, and 15 because of the boys' illnesses. William Wallace Lincoln gradually weakened and died about 5:00 P.M. on February 20.[11]

Although virtually everyone agrees that Willie Lincoln was sick for nearly three weeks before his death, there is little consensus about the nature of his illness. Ruth Painter Randall, in her study *Lincoln's Sons*, lays out various possibilities without really espousing one. Willie could have gotten sick from riding his pony in bad weather, from poor sanitation, or from microbes causing "bilious fever," malaria, or typhoid fever. Others have suggested that Willie died from pneumonia, smallpox, tuberculosis, or congestive heart failure. Several have surmised that Willie's kidneys and heart had been damaged by his bout of scarlet fever in 1860, making him less resistant to the worst aspects of whatever disease he had. Dr. John Sotos, who has fixated on the idea that most members of Lincoln's family suffered from MEN2B and associated cancers, proposed that Willie could have been more susceptible to disease because of this condition.[12]

Several diseases can be dismissed immediately. Smallpox was never mentioned in connection with Willie in sources of the period, nor was tuberculosis, which would have produced other symptoms and probably a longer illness.[13] Willie and Tad would have been unlikely to contract tuberculosis at roughly the same time. Furthermore, Tad ultimately recovered from the illness. Congestive heart failure as a cause of death is associated with the idea that Willie, as well as his father, had the connective tissue disorder Marfan syndrome.[14] Willie's health could well have been weakened by previous illness, but there is no way to know for sure.[15]

"Bilious fever," as used in the nineteenth century, was not a precise term. It could refer to malaria, typhoid, or other fevers that seemed to combine several diseases.[16] Bilious also tended to indicate nausea. While some historians mentioned bilious fever (sometimes as a synonym for malaria) as a possibility, more focused on malaria specifically as the cause of Willie's death.[17] As mentioned previously, malaria is spread by female anopheles mosquitoes, all of which, by January, would have been killed by the cold weather of a Washington, DC, winter. Once a person has had malaria, he or she retains the parasite in the blood, and attacks can recur when the immune system is disturbed by stress or another illness. Dr. W. A. Evans, writing in 1932, thought that "pernicious malaria," an extremely serious case brought on by a relapse, was the cause of Willie's death. However, there are several problems with this diagnosis. Although, as we have seen earlier, Abraham and Mary both apparently had malaria in Illinois and during the summer or fall of 1861 in Washington, there is no indication that the boys also had malaria. In addition, as author Milton Shutes pointed out, a cold, if Willie had one, was not likely to be a serious enough illness to trigger a malaria relapse.[18] It should also be noted that Tad became ill with the same disease within a week of Willie. A malaria relapse would not be contagious, nor would a second person be likely to have an independent relapse at so coincidental a time.

Shutes himself argued that Willie died of "bronchopneumonia," a disease fairly common in children and a diagnosis that he believed fit with Elizabeth Keckly's descriptions of Willie's illness, such as they were. Several other scholars also favor a pneumonia diagnosis.[19] While pneumonia seems in many ways to be a reasonable cause of Willie's death, there is still the fact that Tad also came down with the disease.

In addition, it is important to consider what people at the time believed Willie had died from. The *Washington National Intelligencer* of February 10, 1862, and the *Washington Chronicle* of February 23 both called Willie's disease "typhoid fever," while the *National Republican* of February 21 described it as "an intermittent fever assuming a typhoid character." Rebecca Pomroy, who came to nurse Tad after Willie's death, said that Tad had typhoid. Shutes discounted typhoid fever as the cause because that disease generally spreads in warmer weather, but a number of historians and other authors have accepted the typhoid fever diagnosis.[20] Typhoid fever may have been more prevalent during the summer, perhaps because the germs are so easily spread by flies. However, typhoid is a disease that can be transmitted by food and water contaminated with infected excrement at any time of the year. Several army camps and hospitals in Washington, DC, had typhoid epidemics that winter, and General George B. McClellan was ill with typhoid from December 23, 1861, to about January 13,

1862. Some have suggested that Willie and Tad were infected by contaminated Potomac River water piped into the White House by the plumbing system. This seems unlikely, because Willie and Tad were the only ones who got sick. However, Willie and Tad, young boys with only limited discipline, tended to get into whatever they could. It would not be surprising if they encountered typhoid bacteria in the reportedly nasty White House basement, a nearby marsh that served as a sewage dump, or one of the army camps they visited. Willie and Tad could have been exposed to typhoid fever at the same time but developed it at different rates, as the incubation period is one to three weeks. Or Tad could have gotten typhoid from Willie if exposed to some of Willie's waste products. Typhoid patients can develop additional complications, such as pneumonia.[21] It is possible that Willie got pneumonia resulting in his death while Tad did not.

Both Abraham and Mary Lincoln were devastated by Willie's death. He was a bright, polite, and compassionate child and allegedly the Lincolns' favorite son. Lincoln wept openly on several occasions and reportedly mourned on Thursdays, the day of Willie's death, for some weeks. But Lincoln had a country in the midst of civil war to manage, and by late March, he appeared to be past the most debilitating aspects of his grief.[22]

Mary's case was much different. She collapsed in hysterical sobbing and took to her bed for some time. Possibly she had a nervous breakdown. Unfortunately, Tad was still extremely ill, possibly fatally so, it seemed at the time. Mary could do nothing to care for him; instead, she needed nursing herself. While Lincoln spent as much time as he could with Tad, especially at night, he had other pressing responsibilities and could not become a full-time nurse. Other friends stepped in to care for Tad or watch him at night, including Illinois senator Orville H. Browning and his wife, Eliza, as well as Julia Bates, wife of the attorney general. Mary Jane Welles, wife of the secretary of the navy, cared for Mary, as did Mary's sister Elizabeth Edwards, who arrived from Springfield on February 25. On February 19, Dorothea Dix, the controversial director of the department to provide women nurses for the hospitals, had offered Lincoln a nurse to help with Willie. At that time, he politely declined, but he soon requested someone to care for Tad. Dix sent Rebecca Pomroy, a Massachusetts widow who had been nursing soldiers at the Columbian College Hospital on the edge of Washington, DC.[23]

Pomroy was evidently an encouragement to Tad as well as to his parents. In fact, at first, Tad wanted no one to care for him besides Pomroy and his father. A devout Christian who had experienced the loss of her own husband, two children, and two siblings, Pomroy brought a hard-won sense of serenity and trust in God that impressed and influenced both Lincoln and Mary, although Pomroy probably had a greater effect on Lincoln. Mary, instead, came to believe the ideas of the Spiritualists and drew comfort from allegedly communicating with Willie by herself and through mediums.

As Tad and Mary recovered during March, Pomroy seems to have split her time between the White House and the Columbian College Hospital. Even after the Lincolns no longer needed her services, they encouraged Pomroy to visit them and to stay at the White House for rest and relaxation; they also gave her flowers and treats for the men at the hospital.[24]

Although a Washington, DC, newspaper reported that Mary was nearly back to normal health on March 20 and that she received a visitor on March 21, she remained emotionally fragile for months. The mention of Willie's name, or anything that reminded her of him, would cause an emotional episode. Mary gave away all his toys and other belongings. She refused to let Bud and Holly Taft, the Lincoln boys' best friends, ever come to the White House again, even though it meant that Tad also lost his playmates as well as his brother. The effects of Mary's grief went beyond her immediate family and friends. During the summer, she would not allow the Marine Band to give weekly concerts on the White House grounds, as they usually did. Finally, in mid-July, Mary spent some time in New York and Boston because, as she wrote a friend, "a removal from the scene of our misery was found very necessary."[25]

Tad was no longer considered to be critically ill by February 26, but his recovery was slow. His aunt Elizabeth Edwards told her daughter Julia on March 1 that "Tad is still feeble, can merely walk a few steps at a time." The next day she reported that Tad "is very prostrated with his illness, and saddened with the loss, he evidently suffers from, yet permits no allusion to. . . . We consider Tad quite out of danger, even convalescent, but still unable to sit up." Lincoln wrote Tad a five dollar check on March 10, to be cashed "when he is well enough to present," apparently part of an effort to help Tad recover.[26]

Senator Browning, who had been so helpful to the Lincolns in the immediate aftermath of Willie's death, continued to visit the White House with some frequency. On April 10, Browning found that Lincoln was sick in bed and so did not get to see the president until evening. After Lincoln had been out for a ride, he was "comfortable and in very good spirits." The two men visited for at least an hour. On April 25, Lincoln had a headache in the evening, so the men relaxed, reading and talking about poetry. Lincoln also had a headache on the evening of May 2, when he and Browning spent an hour together.[27]

Dr. Henry W. Bellows, a Unitarian minister and the president of the United States Sanitary Commission, visited Lincoln with several other commission leaders about commission business on April 19. Among other things, Bellows "advised him to take his meals at regular hours. His health was so important to the country." Lincoln replied, "Well, I cannot take my vittles regular. I kind o' just browse around." Technically, Lincoln did have a meal schedule: breakfast at 9:00 A.M., lunch at 2:00 P.M., and dinner at 6:00 P.M., but he frequently ignored it. His secretary John Hay reported that Lincoln usually had a breakfast of "an egg, a piece of toast," and coffee. Generally, lunch consisted of a biscuit and milk in the winter and a biscuit and grapes or other fruit during the summer. Hay remarked that Lincoln "was very abstemious—ate less than any one I know. Drank nothing but water—not from principle, but because he did not like wine or spirits." Artist Francis Carpenter, who lived in the White House for six months while painting a picture of Lincoln and his cabinet at the first reading of a draft of the Emancipation Proclamation, confirmed reports of Lincoln's irregular eating and sleeping habits. When Mary was away, Lincoln tended to forget about food unless he was hungry or the servants insisted that he eat. Sometimes he had meals brought to his office. In general, Lincoln never paid much attention to food.[28] This may have affected his health, or at least his energy level.

On Monday evening, May 5, 1862, along with Secretary of War
Edwin M. Stanton and Secretary of the Treasury Salmon P. Chase,
Lincoln left Washington on the revenue ship *Miami* for Fortress
Monroe, Virginia. That Tuesday, Lincoln tried to eat lunch aboard
ship, but the seas were rough and "the President gave it up almost
as soon as he began, & declaring himself too uncomfortable to eat,
stretched himself at length on the locker." Evidently Lincoln was not
an especially good sailor, as he was later reported to be seasick on the
way to City Point on June 20, 1864, as well.[29]

Lincoln was busy during the summer of 1862 and often under a
great deal of pressure. On July 5, he was so exhausted that he went
to bed early. He often had sleepless nights. When Browning stopped
to visit Lincoln on the morning of July 15, he found Lincoln writing
in the library, appearing "weary, care-worn and troubled." When
Browning inquired how he was, Lincoln replied, "Tolerably well."
Browning told Lincoln that he "regretted that troubles crowded so
heavily upon him, and feared his health was suffering. He held me by
the hand, pressed it, and said in a very tender and touching tone—
'Browning I must die sometime.'" Browning reminded Lincoln how
closely he was connected to the well-being of the country, "and disaster to one would be disaster to the other, and I hope you will do all
you can to preserve your health and life."[30] It is not surprising that
Lincoln suffered periods of depression during the Civil War, given
the continual stresses of his position.

As fall approached, Lincoln apparently felt poorly on September
8. He sprained his wrist on the morning of September 13 trying to
rein in his horse, which was running out of control on the way to
the White House from the Soldiers' Home, where the president and
his family lived during the summer. Evidently the wrist still bothered him on September 25, as Dr. Isachar Zacharie treated Lincoln's
sprain that day. Three days earlier, Lincoln had written a testimonial
commending Zacharie's successful treatment of Lincoln's foot problems.[31] Sometime in 1862, Lincoln also had a terrible toothache, and
Dr. G. S. Wolf extracted the problem tooth for him. According to
Milton Shutes, Lincoln showed up at Wolf's office with a little bottle
of chloroform and took several deep whiffs of it to ease the pain.[32]

When the newspaper reporter Noah Brooks, who had known Lincoln in Springfield, saw the president in Washington in December 1862, he was shocked at the changes in Lincoln's appearance. His eyes seemed to have lost their light, to be sunken, and to have a "far-away look." Lincoln's face was "drawn" and "pale and colorless," with "an air of profound sadness." Benjamin B. French, the commissioner of public buildings, had many occasions to see the Lincolns, as he was involved in arrangements for public functions such as receptions. He spent about a half hour with Lincoln on February 18, 1863, and noted, "He certainly is growing feeble. He wrote a note while I was present, and his hand trembled as I never saw it before, and he looked worn & haggard."[33] Although it is not known what Lincoln's physical problem was at that time, it could have been exacerbated by the approaching anniversary of Willie's death on February 20. Certainly Lincoln was not ill all the time, as on March 3 French reported that Lincoln "looked better than I ever saw him before at a reception." Nevertheless, naval officer John A. Dahlgren found Lincoln appearing "thin and badly—is very nervous and complains of everything" when the president visited the Navy Department on March 29.[34]

Lincoln, Mary, and Tad went to visit General Joseph Hooker in Virginia April 4–10, 1863. When someone mentioned to Lincoln that the rest would be good for him, he replied, "I suppose it is good for the body. But the tired part of me is inside and out of reach." Mary went to Philadelphia in mid-June, where she had some sort of "indisposition." Lincoln sent her several telegrams to let her know that he was well. French reported that the morning of June 17, Lincoln "was in excellent spirits. I wonder whether he ever has a moment of leisure when he is awake! I should think this constant toil and moil would kill him."[35]

On July 2, Mary left the Soldiers' Home in the Lincolns' carriage on her way to the White House. About 10:00 A.M., as the carriage neared Mount Pleasant Hospital, the driver's seat became detached from the carriage, and he and the seat fell off. Evidently someone had removed the screws that fastened the seat in what may have been sabotage directed against Lincoln. The horses spooked, and Mary jumped from the out-of-control carriage. She fell when landing and gashed the back of her head on a stone, receiving some bruises but having no broken bones. Doctors from the hospital treated her and sent her on to the Soldiers' Home or the White House. Mary did well for several days. In fact, Lincoln telegraphed Robert, "Don't be uneasy. Your mother very slightly hurt by her fall." However, infection set in, and Mary became seriously ill. Lincoln hired Rebecca Pomroy again, who cared for Mary for three weeks. By July 28, Mary was sufficiently recovered to travel with Robert and Tad to the White Mountains of New Hampshire for further convalescence. Robert later believed that Mary never fully recovered from the effects of this accident.[36]

On July 22, before Mary left for the north, Lincoln was very unwell in the morning and ate almost nothing all day. However, while his wife was gone, Lincoln sent periodic telegrams to let her know that he was well. Toward the end of her stay, Mary caught a bad cold and was anxious to return to Washington, but she wanted to make sure that the malaria season was over. She and Tad finally got back on September 28.[37]

About mid-November, Tad Lincoln became sick, an occurrence that, given their previous experiences with Eddie and Willie, was very alarming to his parents. It is not clear when Tad became ill, how long he was sick, or what he had. The first indication of his illness in any surviving source is that on November 18, Tad was too ill to eat his breakfast, which depressed his father and made his mother hysterical. Because Lincoln was leaving by train at noon in order to attend the Gettysburg Cemetery dedication the following day, the stress increased. Mary telegraphed Lincoln after the doctor had visited Tad that evening that "we hope dear Taddie is slightly better." On November 20, Lincoln reported to Edward Everett, who had been the main speaker at Gettysburg the previous day, that Tad "we hope is past the worst." The most common diagnosis is that Tad had "scarletina" (scarlet fever), although several have suggested that Tad had varioloid (mild smallpox) or even regular smallpox and was the source of his father's subsequent infection. In that case, Tad would have to have been sick for quite awhile before November 18, since the incubation period for smallpox is generally seven to seventeen days and the person with smallpox is usually most contagious beginning about the fourth day of illness. The *Washington Chronicle* reported that Tad, after a lengthy bout with scarlatina, was much better as of November 27.[38]

Meanwhile, Lincoln, on his way to Gettysburg on November 18, reportedly told his secretary John Hay that he felt weak. The next morning, Lincoln remarked to secretary John Nicolay that he felt dizzy; however, Lincoln performed all his ceremonial responsibilities. That evening, on the way back to Washington on the train, Lincoln was feeling quite unwell with a severe headache and fever. He lay down with a wet towel on his face and was cared for by his sometime valet William Johnson, a black man who had come with him from Springfield to Washington. Back in the capital, although not very well, Lincoln continued to do at least some work for the next few days and to see some people. However, on November 25, he was sick enough to go to bed and stay there. On November 27, Lincoln's doctor ordered that the president was not to have visitors, and Lincoln canceled a meeting with his cabinet.[39]

By November 30, although still in bed, Lincoln was able to work on his annual message to Congress, due when the legislators convened in early December. Still confined to his room, Lincoln was recovering enough to see Benjamin B. French on government business on December 2. Apparently Mary considered Lincoln nearly recovered, since on December 3 she left for a week in New York, where she arrived that evening tired and headachy. The Lincolns exchanged a number of telegrams during her absence, in which he always reassured her, "All doing well." In the various telegrams that the Lincolns sent at any time when they were absent from each other, Mary frequently mentioned her own ailments, but Lincoln always indicated that he was doing well. Whether he actually was always well is a question that cannot be answered. By December 10, Lincoln was seeing some visitors and attending to some business. He may have overdone it, for on December 12, he was too unwell to receive callers. A sure sign of his recovery was attending a play at Ford's Theatre with his family on December 14. At the cabinet meeting the following day, Secretary of the Navy Gideon Welles reported that "the President was well and in fine spirits." At this point, Lincoln could be considered recovered, although the process of fully regaining his strength may have continued for some time.[40]

It is not entirely clear when Lincoln was diagnosed with "varioloid," a mild form of smallpox most likely to be contracted by someone who had been vaccinated or had had smallpox before. Lincoln is not known to have had either a vaccination or a previous case. At least some sources suggest the diagnosis came on November 21, the point at which Lincoln allegedly joked to those who were always seeking favors, "Now I have something I can give everybody." (Several men's diary entries indicate that the joke was receiving its greatest publicity around December 19.) At any rate, William O. Stoddard, one of Lincoln's secretaries, reported that after the diagnosis, Lincoln's doctor vaccinated all the White House staff and residents. No one else at the White House is known to have gotten the disease except William Johnson, whose severe illness ended fatally. There was a widespread smallpox epidemic in Washington at the time, however, so both Lincoln and Johnson could have gotten the disease anywhere. Some doctors have questioned whether Lincoln really had varioloid or whether he was suffering from full-blown smallpox that his doctors called varioloid in order to reassure people. Researchers Armond S. Goldman and Frank C. Schmalstieg analyzed all of Lincoln's symptoms that they could find described in any source and compared them in a handy table with standard symptoms of smallpox, chicken pox, herpes, and Rocky Mountain spotted fever. They concluded that Lincoln had had regular smallpox rather than a milder form. Whatever form of the illness he had, Lincoln apparently did not suffer significant permanent health damage as a result.[41]

Noah Brooks, newspaper correspondent for the *Sacramento Daily Union*, attended the White House reception on New Year's Day 1864. He reported to his paper, "The President looks better since he has had the varioloid. I don't mean to insinuate that the disease has added any new charms to his features; but his complexion is clearer, his eyes less lack-luster and he has a hue of health to which he has long been a stranger." Lincoln seems, from various reports, to have remained healthy into early February.[42]

On February 13, Lincoln managed to attend a reception but afterward reported to Salmon P. Chase, who wanted to see him, "I am unwell, even now, and shall be worse this afternoon." When Lincoln tried to meet with Chase two days later, the treasury secretary was out sick. Lincoln was apparently either not really well on the fifteenth or got sick again, as Mary reported to General Daniel Sickles that Lincoln was "a little better to day" on February 20. She planned to "try & persuade him, to take some medicine & rest a little on the morrow." She then invited Sickles to dinner on February 21. French noted that Lincoln was well and very cheerful at White House receptions on March 23 and April 2. In fact, on the twenty-third he was "as full of fun and story as I ever saw him."[43]

The Lincolns were planning a trip to Fortress Monroe, Virginia, in April, but on April 11, Lincoln wrote to General Benjamin F. Butler canceling the visit because Mary was "so unwell." Evidently it was not one of her usual migraines but something contagious, for on April 16, a local newspaper reported Lincoln to be "quite indisposed" and not receiving visitors. By April 28, Mary was again in New York, and Lincoln telegraphed that he was "very well." On May 26, Mary had a "bilious headache." Lincoln sent Dr. Stone a request for a prescription for her. The following day, Mary wrote a note to her friend Mary Jane Welles, giving more detail than usual about her problem. "I was quite unable during several hours yesterday to leave my bed, owing to an intensely severe headache & although it has left me, yet I am feeling so weak this morning that I fear, that I shall be prevented from visiting the hospitals today." She proposed making the visit on Monday. Mary continued, "I believe, you are likewise, a sufferer, from these bilious attacks & know how much inclined to *nausea* they leave you."[44]

On June 20, Lincoln and Tad left for City Point, Virginia, to visit Ulysses S. Grant and the Army of the Potomac. Although Lincoln was seasick on the way down, he returned to Washington on June 23 "sunburned and tired, but refreshed and cheered," according to John Hay. Lincoln was "slightly indisposed" on June 28 but attended the cabinet meeting nevertheless. Although there are few specific comments about Lincoln family illnesses during the summer and fall of

1864, in early September a disaster was narrowly averted. Benjamin B. French reported on September 9 that he was "at the President's all the morning with some gasfitters, trying to find a leak of gas, which almost suffocated the President in his own office!" Mary had an "intense headache" July 19 and "a little tedious indisposition" in mid-September. The Lincolns were temporarily concerned about Robert's health in mid-October, although no specific information now survives about whatever ailed him.[45]

French recorded in his diary that at the January 21, 1865, White House reception, Lincoln "appeared well and in excellent spirits, and Mrs. Lincoln never appeared better," being cheerful and kind to each guest. Yet there is an overwhelming collection of opinion indicating that in early 1865, Lincoln really was not well. According to Milton Shutes (who does not indicate his sources), Dr. Stone kept warning Lincoln that he was nearing nervous exhaustion. On February 6, James Speed, who had become attorney general in December 1864, came to see Lincoln, angry because of the number of pardons Lincoln was granting. When Lincoln rose quickly in protest, he fainted. Stone ordered Lincoln kept in bed for at least twenty-four hours. When Browning stopped to see Lincoln on the evening of February 23, he found that "the President looked badly and felt badly—apparently more depressed than I have seen him since he became President." About this same time, Lincoln had a visit with his old friend Joshua Speed. Less than a year later, Speed reported to Herndon that Lincoln had admitted health problems. "I am said he very unwell—my feet & hands are always cold—I suppose I ought to be in bed."[46]

Mary also reported an incident to the journalist and reformer Jane Grey Swisshelm just before the president's widow left Washington for Chicago after Lincoln's death. Mary related that shortly before Lincoln's second inauguration, he had not been feeling well and so had sent for some "blue pills" (calomel) from the pharmacy where David Herold (later discovered to be one of the assassination conspirators) worked. Lincoln took the pills before bed, as usual. However, the next morning his face was as white as a pillowcase, and he was unable to get out of bed. Lincoln was anxious to be up because he had so much to do, but Mary insisted that he stay in bed, and he was really too weak to do otherwise. Recovery took several days. Lincoln and Mary "both thought it so strange that the pills should affect him in that way; they never had done so before, and both concluded they would get no more medicine there, as the attendant evidently did not understand making up prescriptions." Mary had never considered that it might be a case of deliberate poisoning before her conversation with Swisshelm. Historians, of course, have no way of knowing whether the medicine was poisoned or there was some other error in compounding the preparation.[47]

On March 4, 1865, Abraham Lincoln was inaugurated for his second term as president of the United States. It was a solemn occasion in many respects. The terrible war was still going on, although probably winding down. The matter of how best to reconstruct the states after the conflict had to be determined. Lincoln already knew, from his wartime attempts, that Reconstruction would not be easy. Other people, including many congressmen and senators, thought they knew better than Lincoln what should be done. Lincoln had just taken on a very heavy burden for four more years. He had no illusions. It is probably not surprising that he seemed depressed, tired, and ill. He would have no real respite, even when the war ended.

Lincoln was sick in mid-March, sick enough not to see visitors on March 13 and to hold the cabinet meeting in his bedroom on March 14. While back in his office on the fifteenth, he saw only the cabinet and a few others on important matters and was still rather weak on the sixteenth.[48]

Previous visits to the army had provided a change of scene for Lincoln, so at General Grant's invitation, Lincoln and his family departed on the *River Queen* for City Point on March 23. Mary, in a note to Senator Charles Sumner as they were about to leave, remarked, "I cannot but devoutly hope, that change of air & rest may have a beneficial effect on my good Husband's health." Gideon Welles assessed Lincoln's situation in his diary that day: "The President has gone to the front, partly to get rid of the throng that is pressing upon him, though there are speculations of a different character. He makes his office more laborious than he should. Does not generalize and takes upon himself questions that properly belong to the Departments, often causing derangement and irregularity. The more he yields, the greater the pressure upon him. It has now become such that he is compelled to flee. There is no doubt he is much worn down."[49]

Unfortunately, the trip did not start out with any advantage to Lincoln's health. He soon became "indisposed." Apparently it was not Lincoln's usual seasickness, but he suspected it was related to the drinking water supplied from the Potomac River at Washington. Mary and Tad seem to have been somewhat ill also. The ship stopped at Fortress Monroe to take on fresh water for Lincoln. Arriving in City Point on the evening of March 24, Lincoln was in good spirits at breakfast the next morning but did not eat much. He went out to the battlefield that afternoon where he saw many dead and wounded, both Union and Confederate, from a fight that morning. Given his general run-down state of health and his illness on the boat, it is hardly surprising that Lincoln "looked worn and haggard" on the way back and declined dinner with General Grant in favor of resting on the *River Queen*. By the next morning, Lincoln was "quite recovered from the fatigue and excitement of the day before."[50]

On March 26, Grant staged a review of the troops for Lincoln and his party. He assigned Horace Porter to escort Mary Lincoln and Julia Grant, bringing them in an army ambulance that had been modified to improve their comfort. Mary, who did not want to be late for the review, urged the driver to go faster over the rough roads. The improved springs bounced the passengers higher than usual, and Mary hit her head on the roof, triggering a migraine. Mary became upset, berating Mrs. Grant, Lincoln, the wife of General E. O. C. Ord, and just about everyone in range. Mortified after her uncontrolled temper fit, Mary remained "indisposed," in seclusion, for most of the next several days aboard the *River Queen* before departing for Washington on April 1, leaving Lincoln and Tad behind. While they were separated, Lincoln sent Mary numerous telegrams and assured her that his health was improving. Mary returned to City Point again on April 6 for the last several days of the visit.[51]

Meanwhile, Lincoln had quite a busy schedule. With the fall of Petersburg and then Richmond, Lincoln had an opportunity to visit both places. John S. Barnes, commander of the USS *Bat*, which served as the escort ship for the *River Queen*, accompanied Lincoln on many of his activities. Barnes noted that Lincoln did not seem tired by his trip to Petersburg on April 3, but the visit to Richmond the next day was much more strenuous, including a walk surrounded by crowds of newly freed people. When he got to the Confederate White House, he sat down in Jefferson Davis's office chair. Lincoln "was pale and haggard, and seemed utterly worn out with fatigue and the excitement of the past hour." He asked for a drink of water and wanted to rest.[52]

On Friday, April 8, Lincoln made a marathon visit to the hospitals of each corps of Grant's army. During the visit, which lasted more than five hours, he shook the hand of and spoke to each patient, whether convalescent or seriously ill. He made sure to visit the Confederate prisoners among the patients and went back to go through a ward that had been missed. The surgeon who accompanied him was concerned that after shaking more than 5,000 hands, Lincoln would have a lame arm. To demonstrate that this was not so, Lincoln picked up an ax and vigorously chopped some wood. According to Francis Carpenter, who was not there, Lincoln then extended the ax horizontally with his outstretched right arm. There he held the ax without quivering, a feat no one else present could match. However, when Lincoln returned to the boat, he admitted to Mary that he was very tired from shaking hands and would have liked to go to bed immediately. Later that night, Lincoln and his party left for the return trip to Washington.[53]

The party arrived in Washington on the evening of April 9. The following day, Gideon Welles noted that Lincoln was "looking well and feeling well." Mary remarked to Charles Sumner on April 11 that Lincoln was feeling better. His "pilgrimage through the hospitals, although a labor of love, to him, fatigued him very much." Lincoln had "quite a severe headache" again on April 13.[54]

As the Lincolns went to Ford's Theatre for a little relaxation on April 14, what was the state of the president's health? Clearly, he had been worn down by the overwhelming pressures of leading the country during four years of devastating civil war. People commented about his physical changes, and photos showed the facial effects of aging. Lincoln also had several illnesses during the previous months.

A few days away at City Point with Grant and his army had provided a change of scenery but not necessarily real rest or relaxation of stress. The visit had probably not made any significant difference with his headaches, for Lincoln suffered a severe one within days of his return. Yet Lincoln's physical situation does not appear to have been dire or unrelieved decline. While on some days he tired easily, not necessarily surprising after his recent illness, on others Lincoln displayed true feats of strength and endurance.

A number of medical doctors have questioned whether Lincoln's physical decline can be attributed solely to stress and routine illnesses. They, and some historians, have theorized about a variety of possible conditions that they believe could have led to Lincoln's deterioration.

LINCOLN AND THE MEDICAL
BANDWAGON

I n the late 1960s, when the author's younger sister was diagnosed with a congenital heart arrhythmia, one of the first things that the doctor told the family was that Winston Churchill had also suffered from this problem. Evidently, many believe that it comforts a patient to know that others have lived famously productive lives while suffering from the same physical condition. This seems to be especially true when Abraham Lincoln is the sufferer to whom the patient can be compared.

Over the course of time, an increasing number of conditions and diseases have been attributed to Lincoln, including (alphabetically) aortic regurgitation, ataxia, attention deficit disorder, cancer, cardiac insufficiency, congestive heart failure, crossed eyes, depression, epilepsy, homosexuality, hypogonadism, Marfan syndrome, MEN2B, mercury poisoning, syphilis, thyroid problems, and tuberculosis. Obviously, Lincoln could not have had all the diseases alleged and survived to be assassinated.[1]

As anyone who has ever gone to the doctor with mysterious aches and pains knows, it can be hard for medical professionals to diagnose a patient in person, even with many elaborate tests. It should not be surprising, therefore, that it is extremely difficult to determine the illnesses of people who lived in the mid-nineteenth century and whose ailments were described only in a sketchy manner by casual observers. A number of doctors, historians, and other interested persons have made valiant attempts to diagnose Lincoln, often stimulated by recent advances in medical knowledge. Some of these attempts have provoked considerable controversy, and few have led to any real consensus.

Abraham Lincoln *may* have been dying in early 1865. Had he not been assassinated, he could have died from aortic insufficiency or congestive heart failure, caused by Marfan syndrome, before the end of his second term as president, as several doctors have proposed. Marfan syndrome seems to be the earliest, and one of the most tenacious, of the "bandwagon" medical issues associated with Lincoln.

In 1896, Antoine Bernard-Jean Marfan, a Parisian pediatrician, was the first to publish a case history of a patient with the syndrome. The disease involves a person's connective tissue, especially in the arms and legs, eyes, and heart. A person who has Marfan syndrome is likely to have very long, thin, and rather weak arms and legs, with large hands and feet, long, spidery fingers, and long toes. This person may also have eye problems, especially with the lenses becoming dislocated. In addition, serious heart problems involving valves and the aorta, which may weaken and rupture suddenly and fatally, are characteristic of Marfan syndrome. As a result, persons with untreated Marfan syndrome often die young.[2]

These symptoms are caused by a disorder in a particular gene that controls the production of the protein fibrillin-1, a substance important to connective tissue. Most people inherit Marfan syndrome from their parents, although about 25 percent of cases result from a spontaneous mutation at conception. A person who has the syndrome is always born with it, even if it is not diagnosed until many years later. Although a particular gene is always affected, it is affected in different ways. As a result, individuals vary widely in the nature and severity of the symptoms they experience. As of mid-2011, there was still no laboratory test for Marfan syndrome beyond genetic testing for fibrillin-1 abnormalities. Doctors rely on observation as well as the personal and family medical history of the patient.[3]

Abraham M. Gordon, a Cincinnati physician, was the first person to suggest that Lincoln could have had Marfan syndrome. In a 1962 article, Gordon tried to show that "Lincoln exhibited the skeletal derangements classically associated with the Marfan Syndrome"—that is, he was tall and thin with very long arms and legs. Gordon believed Lincoln had inherited the syndrome from his mother's side of the family (the Hankses).[4]

Two years later, Dr. Harold Schwartz also published an article claiming that Lincoln had Marfan syndrome but that it descended through Lincoln's father's side of the family. Schwartz had treated a young boy with the syndrome who was an eighth-generation descendant of Mordecai Lincoln II, great-great-grandfather of the president. One major problem with the connection between these two cases is that there do not appear to be other family members with the condition. Marfan syndrome does not skip generations, even though not every person in the family will inherit it. So there should be other relatives who clearly had the syndrome if it was hereditary.[5] Nonetheless, some historians and doctors promptly espoused the idea that Lincoln had Marfan syndrome and assumed that the diagnosis was conclusive rather than provisional. They even said that Lincoln had passed the syndrome on to all his sons except Robert. Many newspapers and magazines publicized these findings as well.[6]

Several historians and doctors have carefully analyzed reports of Lincoln's physical attributes, photographs, and artifacts and reached other conclusions. Their research has shown that Lincoln probably did not have Marfan syndrome, for a number of reasons. First of all, Lincoln was tall but did not have excessively long, spidery fingers or toes. This is demonstrated by the life casts of Lincoln's hands made during the Civil War by sculptor Leonard Volk and by the tracings of Lincoln's feet prepared for a shoemaker. In addition, while Lincoln was thin, he was also muscular and strong. As a young man, Lincoln wrestled and participated in other strenuous physical activities. Even as president, within a week of his death, Lincoln chopped wood vigorously. Consequently, there is no evidence of the weakness associated with Marfan syndrome.[7]

Lincoln evidently had some eye problems, but they were more likely related to crossed or wandering eyes. There is no evidence of lens dislocation or retinal detachment. In addition, persons with Marfan syndrome are near-sighted. Lincoln was far-sighted, as his eyeglasses indicate. Further, some have suggested that Lincoln was not suffering from the stresses of leading the country during the war.

Rather, they say, his obvious physical deterioration during his last few months was the result of aortic insufficiency or congestive heart failure, most likely associated with Marfan syndrome. They cite Lincoln's complaint to Joshua Speed that his hands and feet were always cold. However, there is no evidence that Lincoln had any of the cardiovascular problems associated with Marfan syndrome, or he would not have been able to exhibit the strength that he did as late as the beginning of April 1865.[8]

Although these arguments showing that Lincoln did not have Marfan syndrome have been available since 1981, the allegations have not died out. Marfan sufferers, of course, want to be associated with Lincoln. However, John K. Lattimer, one of the physicians most connected with disputing Lincoln's Marfan syndrome diagnosis, published an article pointing out the dangers of saying that Lincoln had the syndrome. For those who actually do have Marfan syndrome and its cardiovascular problems, an attempt to copy their hero and engage in some of the physical activities that Lincoln participated in could be dangerous, if not fatal.[9]

If Lincoln did not have Marfan syndrome but looked somewhat like he did ("marfanoid" characteristics), what disease might he have had instead? This is a question, along with why Lincoln's physical condition deteriorated so drastically during the last months of the war, that cardiologist John G. Sotos has sought to answer with voluminous research in the Lincoln sources. Sotos, a "connoisseur of rare ailments," as one journalist called him, rejected the Marfan syndrome diagnosis and replaced it with an even rarer genetic condition known as multiple endocrine neoplasia type 2b (MEN2B for short). He claimed that "MEN2B explains Lincoln's unusual build, some of his physical habits, his constipation, his 'pseudo-depression,' his awful physical deterioration as President, and the tragically early deaths of three of his four sons." Sotos believed that with this disorder, "even if he had not been shot, Lincoln was dying and had only months to live."[10]

MEN2B was first diagnosed around 1965. Persons with this syndrome have a marfanoid body shape (tall and thin) without having the cardiovascular and eye problems of Marfan syndrome. Persons with MEN2B have other difficulties, however. MEN2B involves the overgrowth of long bones (for example, legs) as well as nerve cells in several areas. These overgrown nerve cells form benign lumps on the lips, tongue, and interior of the cheek, as well as in the digestive tract, causing constipation and diarrhea. Most serious of all, in almost all cases MEN2B sufferers contract thyroid cancer, while about half of them also develop cancer of the adrenal glands on the kidneys.[11]

A number of factors, besides Lincoln's slightly marfanoid appearance, combined to convince Sotos that Lincoln had MEN2B. First, Sotos claimed, using several photographs as evidence, that Lincoln and some of his sons had the bumpy lips characteristic of MEN2B. Second, Lincoln had constipation, as several of Herndon's interviewees pointed out. There is no evidence that Lincoln had diarrhea (unless briefly associated with another illness). Sotos admitted that having constipation is not, by itself, proof of MEN2B. Third, Lincoln had a peculiar style of walking, as well as tended to slouch and lounge when seated, which Sotos saw as indicative of low muscle tone associated with MEN2B. In addition, Sotos used computer graphics programs to show that Lincoln's head was asymmetrical. Although he admitted that everyone's head is uneven somehow, and Lincoln's head shape matched those of babies who had lain "too much on their left rear skull," Sotos, nevertheless, tied this trait in with MEN2B.[12]

The biggest issue for Sotos was Lincoln's serious physical decline during his presidency. Evidently, Lincoln lost a good deal of weight, possibly beginning in the campaign and pre-presidential period with the loss of forty pounds between April 1860 and January 1861. Continued weight loss over the course of the war is evident when photographs are compared, and changes are noted in the life masks of April 1860 and February 1865. Although Sotos admitted that Lincoln could have lost weight because of stress, Sotos was convinced that Lincoln was suffering from slow-growing thyroid cancer, with weight loss as its first symptom. He believed that by early 1865, Lincoln also had adrenal cancer, which accounted for his further weight loss, severe headaches, cold hands and feet, and an episode of fainting. Sotos additionally believed that Eddie, Willie, and Tad Lincoln had inherited MEN2B and that Tad actually died in 1871 of thyroid cancer that had spread to his chest, causing the fluid accumulation that Tad's doctors reported.[13]

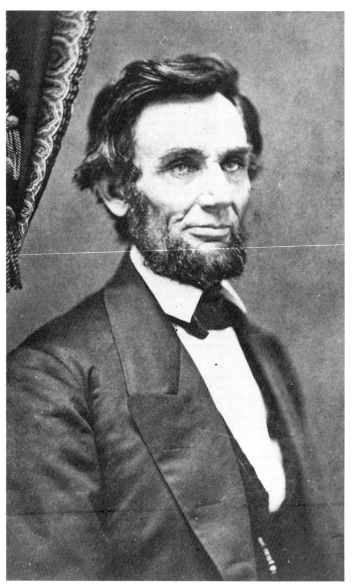

Abraham Lincoln, February 9, 1861. Christopher S. German took this portrait of Lincoln in Springfield just before he left for Washington, DC, to assume the presidency. Library of Congress, LC-USZ62–7334.

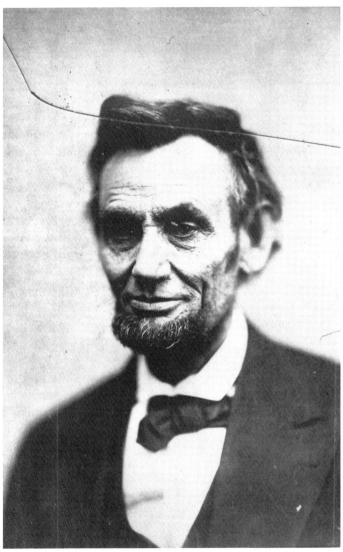

Abraham Lincoln, February 5, 1865. Lincoln clearly had aged during the four years of his presidency. Lincoln fainted the day after the photo session. Taken in Washington, DC, by Alexander Gardner, this image is considered to be Lincoln's last photograph. For many years, historians believed this picture had been taken on April 10, 1865. Library of Congress, LC-USZ62–8812.

Sotos gathered and published a massive amount of material related to the medical status of Lincoln and his family that can be daunting to readers with limited medical backgrounds but can aid researchers. His main problem, however, is his one-track-mind focus on MEN2B. In many cases, Sotos presented other possible explanations for Lincoln's symptoms but inevitably rejected them. Sotos was convinced that Lincoln had the classic symptoms and features of MEN2B. He reasoned that it was better to have one disease fit all categories than to diagnose Lincoln with more than one disease.[14]

There are a number of reasons for treating the MEN2B diagnosis with some skepticism. It is an extremely rare disease. Even though about half the known cases are hereditary, it seems unlikely that Lincoln, three of his sons, and his mother all had it, as Sotos suggested. Although Sotos provided photographic enlargements of the faces of Lincoln, Willie, and Tad, it is difficult for many people to discern most of the facial bumps Sotos noted. In a *Washington Post* interview, Jeffrey E. Moley, a specialist in MEN2B at Washington University School of Medicine in St. Louis, commented after seeing pictures of Lincoln, "The facial appearance is not convincing. Overall, I don't think so," although Moley "would not rule it out completely" because there are always exceptions.[15]

Sotos admitted that "in Lincoln's case, it is too hard to decide whether stress-induced disease or cancer has better support. Both can affect the body widely."[16] Sotos opted to advocate cancer resulting from MEN2B. However, at every level, from newspaper articles and popular magazines to scholarly studies, current media detail the evil effects of continuous stress on the human body. Lincoln certainly qualifies as a person who was under extreme and constant stress for more than four years. It should come as no surprise that he would suffer physical effects. Even presidents who had far fewer strains in office aged noticeably during their term or terms, as can be seen by a comparison of photographs over the course of their presidencies. In addition, Washington, DC, in the 1860s was not exactly a sanitary location. Exposed to various kinds of pollution, as well as to illnesses in hospitals and military camps, Lincoln could have contracted any number of diseases, as he did the smallpox discussed previously. With so many opportunities for multiple illnesses, it seems too convenient that all Lincoln's possible physical ailments should be the result of one rare condition.

One other genetic disease so associated with Abraham Lincoln's family as to sometimes be called "Lincoln's disease" is ataxia. A hereditary condition that involves progressive loss of muscle control, ataxia often initially appears as a staggering walk and slurred speech, as though the person were drunk. There are five types of ataxia caused by different genetic defects. A better case can be made for Lincoln having ataxia than some other diseases. A study of 170 descendants of Lincoln's grandparents Abraham and Bathsheba Herring Lincoln showed 56 of them with spinocerebellar ataxia type 5 (SCA5). More recently, a study of 299 relatives found 129 with a mutant gene and 90 with ataxia symptoms. Nevertheless, Lincoln had only a 25 percent chance of inheriting the disease and is not known to have displayed any of the symptoms, beyond a peculiar sort of walk noted by various people. Because those with the mutant gene can develop ataxia symptoms at virtually any age, researchers suggest that Lincoln could have had SCA5 in its earliest stages.[17]

Ultimately, no one can tell for sure whether Lincoln had Marfan syndrome, MEN2B, or ataxia based on descriptions by his contemporaries. Various researchers, scientists, and curious persons have suggested that DNA testing could prove whether Lincoln had these conditions or not. DNA (deoxyribonucleic acid) is the smaller-than-microscopic series of genetic components from which living beings are made. Humans inherit DNA as part of their chromosomes from both parents. DNA can be tested (through processes too detailed to be described here) to identify individuals, confirm parentage, provide evidence to convict criminals, and, in some cases, pinpoint disease. In many ways, DNA testing may seem like a magic process that can conclusively answer any identity question. However, there are many potential problems with DNA testing that may lower its value in any given case.[18]

There are two kinds of DNA, nuclear and mitochondrial. Nuclear DNA is found in cell nuclei in all of the chromosomes; is passed on to a person, half from each parent; and determines a person's physical characteristics. Mitochondrial DNA controls enzymes that provide energy for the cells. It is shaped differently from nuclear DNA, is inherited entirely from one's mother, and may have as many as thousands of copies in one cell, rather than one or two. DNA begins to deteriorate when a person dies or the cells bearing DNA are separated from the person. Under proper temperature and humidity conditions, some DNA can remain testable for years, even centuries. Unfortunately for Lincoln studies, the DNA that usually survives best is mitochondrial DNA, which does not contain information on the target genetic diseases.[19]

Those who wish to test Lincoln's DNA have a very limited number of specimens to work with. Four institutions have potentially testable material. The Chicago History Museum owns the bed where Lincoln died, the mattress from that bed, and the bloodstained bottom sheet. The National Museum of Health and Medicine in Washington, DC, holds seven skull fragments and a lock of hair from around Lincoln's wound, collected during his autopsy, as well as the bloodstained shirt cuffs of Edward Curtis, one of the physicians who performed the autopsy. Lincoln's suit and the overcoat he was wearing when he was assassinated, along with two pillows from his deathbed and some bloodstained towel fragments, are at Ford's Theatre, owned by the National Park Service. Finally, there is a small strip of bloody pillowcase at the Grand Army of the Republic Museum in Philadelphia. While there are a few other odds and ends of supposed Lincoln biological matter in other museums and private collections, the Lincoln specimens remain very limited. Furthermore, as a result of an attempt to steal Lincoln's body in 1876, he now rests beneath tons of concrete, making any possibility of exhuming him highly unlikely. Just because various museums have Lincoln specimens does not mean they are willing to give them up for testing, because all the tests now performable destroy the sample being tested without assuring that useful results can be produced.[20] Each of the diseases under consideration has a number of variations caused by different mutations to the DNA. Initially, scientists were not even sure which chromosomes could be associated with Marfan syndrome, the disease for which testing was first proposed.

In June 1989, Darwin J. Prockop, director and chairman of the Jefferson Institute of Molecular Medicine at Jefferson Medical College of Philadelphia, made a formal proposal to the National Museum of Health and Medicine to test some of its Lincoln autopsy materials. Prockop and his associates wanted washings from the roots of Lincoln's hair and one milligram of bone to establish "a genetic library of Lincoln's genome" and test for DNA showing that Lincoln had Marfan syndrome. The museum's response was very cautious because its officials realized they would be setting a precedent if they permitted destructive medical testing of historical specimens.[21]

The museum took two steps. On February 9, 1991, its officials held a symposium in Washington, DC, on Lincoln's health. They then convened a panel of nine experts on May 1, 1991, to examine the issues. The panel consisted of two museum managers, the president of the National Marfan Foundation, five physicians (two of whom were geneticists), and one Lincoln historian (Cullom Davis, then head of the Lincoln Legal Papers); it was chaired by Victor McKusick, a medical genetics professor. They had four questions to answer pertaining to the "ethical, legal and social implications of conducting genetic tests on human medical specimens." The panel concluded that the proposal was scholarly, appropriate, and historically interesting but not vitally important. The experts believed Lincoln probably would have agreed to the testing because he was interested in science and technology. They did not think testing would be a violation of Lincoln's privacy because by that time he had been dead for 126 years and had no living descendants. In addition, Lincoln's blood had already been typed and his specimens had been on display for years. They also believed that it was acceptable for a tiny amount of material to be carefully tested, even if the testing destroyed it.[22]

A second panel of physicians met April 14 and 15, 1992. Also headed by McKusick, this group was less optimistic, pointing out the likelihood that the specimens would have only mitochondrial DNA and were probably contaminated from poor handling over the years. They were also concerned whether there was even an accurate way to test DNA for Marfan syndrome. As a result, the Lincoln specimens were not tested in the 1990s.[23]

John G. Sotos raised the idea of DNA testing again in the spring of 2009, this time to test not only for Marfan syndrome but to see if Lincoln had MEN2B. By this point, the National Museum of Health and Medicine, the National Park Service, and the Chicago History Museum had all established policies prohibiting destructive testing on nonrenewable historical specimens. This left the pillowcase fragment at the Grand Army of the Republic Museum in Philadelphia. After much disagreement, at a meeting on May 4, 2009, the museum board rejected the request for DNA testing because members did not "want to take the chance of losing the artifact."[24]

Nevertheless, Sotos was able to find a family who allegedly held a piece of the actress Laura Keene's bloodstained dress and a collector with some Lincoln hair and a piece of bandage. Sotos had these artifacts tested at laboratories in Cleveland, Ohio, and in New Zealand. The suspense of the process was filmed and aired as a National Geographic television special on February 21, 2011. While the laboratories were able to isolate a little DNA on several samples, the results showed no MEN2B. Sotos planned to persevere in his quest on the assumption that it was not really Lincoln's blood on the artifacts, the samples had been contaminated, or they had deteriorated too far to give accurate results.[25]

On April 8, 2011, a Lincoln Biohistory Study Group met at the Chicago History Museum. The group consisted of physicians, geneticists, historians, legal experts, scientists from medical companies, and representatives of associations for the diseases Lincoln may have suffered from. The group heard presentations on what testing had been done already as well as on what might be achieved through further testing. By this time, swabs and samples from Lincoln's deathbed, a bedsheet, the Philadelphia museum pillowcase, and Lincoln's hair had been tested. Only the bedsheet tested positive for DNA but had not been further analyzed. The Ethics Panel subgroup met three more times by teleconference, debating the purposes of such research and whether it could even be justified.[26]

Opinion remains divided on whether to test Lincoln's DNA further. On the one side are those with scientific or personal curiosity, as well as persons who want to see Lincoln as an encouragement and inspiration to fellow sufferers of any condition the president may have had. On the other side are those who wish to preserve rare, nonrenewable historical materials from destruction, plus those who want to protect Lincoln's privacy. The preservationists are especially concerned because the specimens may not have enough proper DNA to test, or they may be contaminated by the DNA of other people who touched them or even sneezed on them, but there is no way to find out without destroying the material in the testing process. (It is rather unnerving to watch the snipping of cloth to be tested during the National Geographic program.) In at least some cases, the proper DNA marker for the disease is uncertain, so the test might be useless. In fact, the testing so far done proves these concerns are justified. Very little DNA has been found, researchers cannot tell to whom it belonged, and it has shown no evidence of the target diseases. Given the relatively recent public interest of Sotos in MEN2B, it would hardly be surprising if in a few years someone else wanted to test for yet another disease. Material needs to be retained for further research. The technology of DNA testing continues to change rapidly. It is entirely possible that a nondestructive test may be developed that would permit both investigation and preservation if the researchers can be patient.

Although homosexuality is not a disease, it has become one of the top medically related controversies of the past several decades in Lincoln studies. As a number of historians have pointed out, there was no indication during Lincoln's lifetime that anyone suspected him of being a homosexual. One noted, "In the 1858 debates Stephen A. Douglas called Lincoln a saloonkeeper, drunkard, ruffian, gambler and betrayer of American troops fighting in Mexico. He certainly would have brought Lincoln's gayness to public attention had such rumor existed." There were contemporary speculations about other public figures, such as James Buchanan, but not about Lincoln.[27]

   According to C. A. Tripp, whose 2005 book, *The Intimate World of Abraham Lincoln*, provided the most extensive presentation of Lincoln as a homosexual, there was little attention to Lincoln's sexual orientation until quite recently. Only Ida Tarbell, Carl Sandburg,

Robert Kincaid, and Margaret Leech earlier in the twentieth century made passing allusions to what Tripp interpreted as Lincoln's homosexual aspects. Otherwise, Tripp faulted historians for missing the homosexuality he deemed obvious.[28]

The first real attempt to present Lincoln as a homosexual was made by gay liberation activist James Kepner in a privately published article in 1971. Kepner concentrated on the relationship between Lincoln and Joshua Speed, a storekeeper with whom Lincoln shared a bed in Springfield, Illinois, for four years. Material from Kepner's article was apparently recycled by a number of the writers who trumpeted Lincoln's homosexuality in the 1990s.

In 1989, Charles Shively, a University of Massachusetts professor, published a book called *Drum Beats*. It was primarily about Walt Whitman but also contained a chapter on Lincoln. However, because Shively was openly gay and had his book published by a gay press, few outside the gay community paid attention to it. The 1990s brought more media discussion about homosexuality in general. An October 1, 1995, *New York Times* article about Lincoln and Joshua Speed seems to have been one of the main starting points for press discussion of Lincoln as gay.[29]

The most important push for the Lincoln homosexuality agenda came with the announcement in 1999 by Larry Kramer, a noted gay activist and playwright, that Lincoln was gay and that Kramer had a Joshua Speed diary to prove it (although no one else ever saw the supposed diary). When Kramer's theories were summarized by Brian Lamb on C-SPAN's *American Presidents* program, the Lincoln-as-gay idea received tremendous media publicity.[30]

C. A. Tripp was a psychologist and sex researcher who had worked with Alfred Kinsey for a number of years. Tripp died in May 2003, a couple of weeks after he finished writing his book on Lincoln's sexuality but before he could edit it. His background as a sex researcher and not a historian, as well as his own homosexuality, affected Tripp's presentation and interpretation of evidence.[31]

An important example of Tripp's problems with historical methodology and wishful thinking is his treatment of Lincoln's age at puberty. According to a Kinsey study, a man who experienced puberty early was more likely to have more and earlier homosexual experiences and to become a homosexual than a man who matured later. Tripp built a case for Lincoln's early puberty and consequent homosexuality based on a single reference by one man interviewed after Lincoln's death by Lincoln's law partner and biographer William Herndon. David Turnham, who moved to Indiana and became acquainted with Lincoln when Lincoln was about ten, described the boy as "a long tall dangling award drowl [awkward droll] looking boy," as well as "raw boned," "odd and gawky." Turnham also said that Lincoln had "hardly attained" his full height by the time he and his family left Indiana in 1830. Nowhere does this account mention puberty, merely that Lincoln was a tall child who had become a tall adult by the end of his teens. Tripp, however, claimed that Lincoln would have hit puberty before his growth spurt began. Thus, if he was tall at the age of ten, he had experienced puberty while he was only nine. Several historians have taken Tripp to task for this misinterpretation of and overreliance on a single source.[32]

Tripp's determination that Lincoln was "predominantly homosexual, but incidentally heterosexual" was not based on newly discovered materials but on reinterpretation of the same sources used by most historians. Because Tripp was a "sex researcher," "alert to homosexual propositions," he could take what would appear to anyone else to be an innocent statement or action and turn it into a homosexual seduction.[33] For example, in the standard account of Lincoln's arrival in Springfield, Speed invited Lincoln to share his bed upstairs over the store because Lincoln was too poor to afford a set of bedding. Lincoln accepted the offer, took his bags upstairs, and returned, exclaiming, "Well, Speed, I'm moved."[34] As far as Tripp was concerned, "the tale is more than suspect; its details are questionable in the extreme." Tripp believed that something else must have happened because Speed could not have made such a "generous" offer and then allowed Lincoln to find his way upstairs alone. It apparently did not occur to Tripp that Speed may have had other customers in the store. Surely the upstairs was not so large that Lincoln could have gotten lost. Instead, Tripp claimed that Speed and Lincoln began "what was to become *the* major event in Lincoln's private life, an intense and ongoing homosexual relationship with Speed." According to Tripp, Speed's invitation was a homosexual proposition that Lincoln accepted, so Tripp believed it was "necessary to make a few further corrections and additions to Speed's account of their first meeting," since Speed was supposedly hiding his homosexual activities. What Tripp based his elaborations on besides his own imagination and Kinsey sex research is not clear.[35]

Not surprisingly, Tripp alleged that Lincoln had more than one homosexual partner and began the book with an account of Lincoln's sleeping with David Derickson, an officer in Company K, 150th Pennsylvania Infantry, Lincoln's bodyguard regiment in Washington, DC, beginning September 7, 1862. Lincoln was spending the nights at the Soldiers' Home just outside the city during the summer and fall of 1862. While Mary and Tad were in Boston and New York from October 20 to November 27, Lincoln spent some time with Derickson and, according to two accounts, slept with Derickson on one or more occasions, even loaning Derickson a nightshirt. While Tripp alleged that Lincoln and Derickson had clandestine homosexual encounters when Mary was out of town to keep them a secret from her, other researchers have suggested that Lincoln was lonely with Mary and Tad gone and was simply enjoying conversation and company. Martin P. Johnson, in his examination of the Derickson allegations, suggests that what shocked the two people who commented about Lincoln and Derickson was not any possible sexual impropriety but the idea that someone of a lower class should be wearing Lincoln's nightshirt. It was a rank and status issue rather than a question of sexuality.[36]

Tripp was also certain that Lincoln had had a homosexual affair with Billy Greene in New Salem because when Herndon interviewed Greene after Lincoln's death, Greene mentioned meeting Lincoln and noticing his "perfect" thighs. Furthermore, Greene and Lincoln had shared a narrow cot in the store where both worked for eighteen months. It evidently did not occur to Tripp that in that era, young clerks would make do with whatever sleeping arrangements were provided for them. There lies Tripp's major problem. He was so attuned to supposed sexual nuances that he could not grasp the social and cultural norms of the nineteenth-century United States.[37]

Tripp's evidence for Lincoln's series of homosexual liaisons boils down to a few central points on which he elaborated extensively. Lincoln was more comfortable with men than with women, especially eligible women. He married late and had an unpleasant relationship with his wife. Finally, Lincoln frequently slept with other men, both before and after his marriage. As several historians have pointed out, with these criteria, most nineteenth-century men could be classified as gay.[38]

It is important to treat the evidence in the context of nineteenth-century practicality and cultural norms rather than in the light of late-twentieth- and early-twenty-first-century sexual disputes. In the early and mid-nineteenth century, men shared beds with other men (as women did with women) in a variety of situations. Siblings grew up sharing beds. Apprentices, farmhands, and clerks shared beds on a long-term basis. Strangers shared beds in taverns and boardinghouses. Privacy was not important and was not expected. Except among the elite, rooms and beds were often at a premium, and as a consequence, people expected to share. William H. Herndon and Charles Hurst shared a bed in the same room as Lincoln and Speed. On the legal circuit, Leonard Swett frequently slept with Lincoln. Given the option of sharing with the tall, thin Lincoln or the 300-pound David Davis, the choice was obvious, as Swett said himself.[39]

Speed and Lincoln's close relationship was not that unusual at the time. Other major nineteenth-century figures also had extremely close male friends in their young manhood, including Daniel Webster, William H. Seward, Edwin M. Stanton, and Salmon P. Chase, none of whom have been accused of homosexual inclinations. Tripp found part of his "evidence" in the fact that Lincoln and Speed shared a bed for four years, not a brief time. Yet this hardly proves a homosexual relationship. It is more important to consider the advantages of sharing a bed. It saved money, and Lincoln was still paying off his debt from the failed store in New Salem. People rarely moved out by themselves in that era. Instead, single persons generally lived in families, with surrogate families, or with employers or roommates. Living alone was not a goal. Companionship and support were more important.[40]

Finally, during the Civil War, accommodations for the soldiers were based on pairs. Each man received a blanket and, during later campaigns, half a tent. Two men together had two blankets and a tent. Even when they were in large tents, barracks, or other buildings, pairs of men shared blankets and bunks, helping to keep each other warm. In many cases, these men remained paired until one of them became sick or was wounded. The survivor would then have to find another partner.[41]

In short, Lincoln's sharing a bed with Joshua Speed, Billy Greene, David Derickson, Leonard Swett, or any other man was nothing unusual during the period and was not indicative of a homosexual relationship. Lincoln was notoriously non-fussy about his clothing and food. There is no reason to suppose that he would have been fussy about sleeping arrangements.[42]

Several historians have accepted Tripp's ideas in whole or in part. Jean Baker, who wrote the introduction to Tripp's book, noted that "Tripp's notion of factual verification defied the canons of the discipline of history," yet she largely accepted his ideas, with the qualifications that Tripp was too hard on Mary Lincoln (about whom Baker had written a biography) and that Lincoln was more likely bisexual than homosexual. Michael B. Chesson, whose "An Enthusiastic Endorsement" was printed in the back of Tripp's book, supported Tripp's findings but thought that Tripp's case was not conclusive. While Chesson believed the issue ought to be studied further, he thought that it was reasonable that Lincoln was homosexual because Lincoln was "different from most men and he knew it."[43] Perhaps the historian most taken with Tripp's arguments has been William Hanchett, a student of Lincoln's assassination. Hanchett's four-part series in the *Lincoln Herald* ruminated on some aspects of Tripp's evidence, mostly agreeing with and building upon it. In the final installment, Hanchett even proposed that Herndon kept Lincoln's homosexuality secret, recording it only in his now-missing memo books and possibly even inventing and planting testimony about Lincoln's passion for women in order to keep that secret.[44]

More historians have chosen to dispute Tripp's theories, either in book reviews or in other writings on Lincoln controversies. One of the first was Michael Burlingame, who provided the dissenting commentary at the end of Tripp's book. While Burlingame agreed with Tripp that the Lincolns had a terrible marriage, he focused on the evidence that showed Lincoln's interest in and courtship of other women before his marriage. Burlingame believed that Tripp's evidence for Lincoln's homosexuality was very weak.[45]

Edward Blum, reviewing Tripp's book for H-Net, thought that "although Tripp asks provocative questions, he offers few compelling answers." Blum found reading the book "excruciating." Other reviewers pointed out Tripp's sloppy historical methodology, meager evidence, overreliance on Kinsey sexual research, and failure to understand cultural attitudes of the nineteenth century.[46] More than one reviewer discerned a homosexual agenda in Tripp's work, a desire "to validate their own sexual tendencies by claiming that Lincoln shared them" (a desire also shared by their straight opponents, Gerald J. Prokopowicz pointed out). Michael Burlingame phrased the issue sharply: "I don't see how the whole question of Lincoln's gayness would explain anything other than making gay people feel better . . . [a]nd I don't think the function of history is to make people feel good. Celebratory history is propaganda."[47]

Tripp and his supporters have had a tendency to make homosexual mountains out of cultural molehills. No one can say for sure that Lincoln *never* had any sort of homosexual encounter. However, based on available evidence, it is highly unlikely that Lincoln was a long-term practicing homosexual with multiple partners, as Tripp has alleged. Nevertheless, it is important to consider this topic thoroughly because it has received so much exaggerated publicity.[48]

LINCOLN AND MEDICAL MATTERS
DURING THE CIVIL WAR

W hen Abraham Lincoln assumed the presidency on March
4, 1861, he had little experience with medical issues beyond
family illnesses and several legal cases that involved alleged medical malpractice or questions of sanity.[1] Once he became president,
Lincoln, in his role as commander in chief, had overall responsibility for the military, including its medical arm. Practically, however,
the secretary of war and the secretary of the navy, along with their
departments, managed the details of military affairs. Yet, over the
course of the war, Lincoln made certain choices that could, directly
or indirectly, help or hinder the medical care of the troops. The
choices, affected at times by bureaucracy or compassion, generally fit
into three broad areas of interaction with medical personnel, civilian
aid groups, and individual patients.

In 1860, the US Army was more or less prepared to take care
of whatever wounds and illnesses its 16,000 troops suffered with a
department consisting of one surgeon general, thirty surgeons, and
eighty-three assistant surgeons. However, a number of medical officers soon left the army and seceded with their states. Thomas Lawson
had joined the military medical corps during the War of 1812 and
had served as surgeon general since 1836. In no physical condition
to lead the department in wartime, Lawson died of a stroke on May
15, 1861. His replacement, Clement A. Finley, was appointed on the
basis of seniority, not because of any skills or desire to expand the

medical service to meet the needs of the rapidly enlarging army. Lincoln would, of course, have signed the commission of Surgeon General Finley, but, overwhelmed with other things to do at the start of his term and the war, the president would probably have left Finley's selection to the medical bureaucracy. Unfortunately, Finley neglected to order supplies, countermanded the construction of a hospital, and generally tried to save money rather than be prepared to save the sick and wounded. Army medical care was also complicated by split responsibilities. The quartermaster department was to provide construction of facilities, transportation, and equipment, while the subsistence department provided supplies.[2]

The army in all its departments was chaotic and undersupplied in the early months of the war, so it is hardly surprising that the medical department had many difficulties. However, civilians stepped in to try to remedy the situation. Local groups provided food and clothing for soldiers from their area. Larger organizations, such as the United States Sanitary Commission, were formed to provide centralized coordination for the efforts of the local groups, as well as medical supplies and sanitation guidelines that the army medical department was not able to provide.[3]

The Sanitary Commission originated in New York in April 1861 and was based on a concept developed in Great Britain during the Crimean War in the mid-1850s. Because the army and its medical department feared and resented any civilian interference or control, they generally opposed the work of the Sanitary Commission and similar groups, despite the crucial aid the commissions provided to the undersupplied soldiers. Four Sanitary Commission founders met with Lincoln as well as with Secretary of War Simon Cameron, Colonel Robert Wood of the medical department, and other Washington leaders in May 1861 to try to gain some official standing for the commission. After some discouragement, Cameron finally issued an order establishing the commission on June 9, naming certain people to inquire into inspection of new recruits, sanitary conditions of troops and camps, and anything else necessary "to the means of preserving and restoring the health, and of securing the general comfort and efficiency of troops." Finley and Wood opposed the commission.

At first, Lincoln was somewhat reluctant to support the commission as well because he thought it might be "a fifth wheel to the coach," something unnecessary. But the president did sign the order on June 13, noting, "I approve the above." In July 1861, when military officers and the medical department opposed the commission in a bill before Congress, Lincoln supported the commission.[4]

Despite his busy schedule, Lincoln made time to see sanitary commissioners, even if the appointment had to be at 9:00 P.M. On August 2, 1861, he notified General John C. Frémont that Dr. Godfrey Aigner would be coming to Frémont's department to inspect its sanitary conditions on behalf of the commission. On September 30, in response to a request from commission executive secretary Frederick Law Olmsted for the public to supply needed blankets for the soldiers, Lincoln endorsed the Sanitary Commission. He noted that "the Sanitary Commission is doing a work of great humanity and of direct practical value to the nation, in this time of its trial. It is entitled to the gratitude and confidence of the people, and I trust it will be generously supported. There is no agency through which voluntary offerings of patriotism can be more effectively made." This notice of Lincoln's support was published in the *New York Tribune* on October 7, 1861. Yet in the fall of 1861, when the Western Sanitary Commission organized a competing group in St. Louis to care for the needs of western soldiers, Lincoln permitted them to remain independent, against the wishes of the New York–based US Sanitary Commission.[5]

By October 1861, the Sanitary Commission leaders were exasperated with Surgeon General Finley and were agitating for his removal. In a two-hour meeting on October 17, Lincoln accused the commissioners of "wanting to run the machine," a charge they denied. They apparently already had William A. Hammond in mind as a suitable replacement for Finley. However, Hammond did not have appropriate seniority, and Secretary of War Cameron opposed him. The commission advocated appointment based on qualifications rather than on seniority. By January 1862, with the possibility of Congress passing a medical department reform bill, the commissioners urged Lincoln to consult them before making any appointments.[6]

On January 11, 1862, Simon Cameron resigned as secretary of war, a post in which he had proved incompetent. His supremely competent and dedicated successor, Edwin M. Stanton, replaced him on January 15. Stanton's appointment brought a whole new dynamic into Lincoln's relations with the medical department and the surgeon general. A man of irascible temperament with strong grudges, Stanton disliked the Sanitary Commission and its candidate for surgeon general. In the interests of working smoothly with Stanton, whose services as secretary of war Lincoln really needed, the president often allowed Stanton to have his way in matters that affected the medical department.[7]

Surgeon General Finley retired under pressure on April 14, 1862. Two days later, Congress finally passed a bill to reform the army medical department. This bill established several new positions and bypassed the seniority system, opening the way for the appointment of the Sanitary Commission's candidate, William A. Hammond. Hammond, at thirty-three, had eleven years' experience in the army medical service but no seniority because he had briefly left the army to teach at a medical school. Although Lincoln received pressure to appoint Assistant Surgeon General Robert Wood instead, Lincoln ultimately gave in to the urgings of the Sanitary Commission and its supporters. Hammond received his appointment as surgeon general on April 25. Despite the fact that Hammond was highly qualified and made some important improvements in soldier medical care, he quickly made some important enemies as well, including a number of the senior surgeons. Even more important, Hammond's strong personality clashed with Stanton's from the beginning, which limited Hammond's effectiveness and ultimately forced his removal from his post. In August 1863, Stanton ordered Hammond on an inspection tour of western hospital posts and refused to allow him to return to Washington, meanwhile appointing his own personal physician, Joseph K. Barnes, as acting surgeon general. When Hammond requested a court-martial, he received one that was rigged against him. Lasting from January until August 1864, the court-martial found Hammond guilty on various charges pertaining to the purchase of blankets and other supplies.[8]

During this medical department crisis, Lincoln never supported Hammond in any way. Lincoln's response to Stanton's vindictive treatment of Hammond is perhaps understandable if Lincoln wished not to cross Stanton himself. Although the Sanitary Commission defended Hammond specifically to Lincoln, treasurer George T. Strong expected even before the trial began that "we shall fail. Stanton is a strong man. He has made up his mind to commit this injustice, and we can hardly hope to prevent him." In August 1864, when Hammond's wife requested an interview with Lincoln to ask him to listen to some additional evidence, Lincoln endorsed her card, "Under the circumstances, I should prefer not seeing Mrs. Hammond." Lincoln also did not reply to a request for an interview with Hammond himself. On August 18, Lincoln endorsed the court-martial orders: "The record, proceedings, findings, and sentence of the Court in the foregoing case are approved; and it is ordered that Brigadier General William A. Hammond, Surgeon General of the United States Army, be dismissed the service, and be forever disqualified from holding any office of honor, profit, or trust under the government of the United States." It was probably not one of Lincoln's finest moments. Yet in some respects, the end of the conflict between Stanton and Hammond was beneficial to the soldiers. Stanton's crony Barnes, who succeeded Hammond, carried out many of Hammond's plans with Stanton's support.[9]

Lincoln had the opportunity to interact with a number of other medical personnel for a variety of reasons during the Civil War. Many men applied to Lincoln for appointment to a position as surgeon for a particular group or at a certain location. Others applied on behalf of their friends or constituents. Dr. Anthony Dignowitz, a Unionist who had had to leave Texas, was recommended for an appointment by General Don Carlos Buell. On August 29, 1861, Lincoln supported his appointment. A few days later, Lincoln consulted with Senator Zachariah Chandler of Michigan about a Dr. William Brodie of Detroit, who seemed well qualified for an appointment but was opposed by Chandler. In most cases, Lincoln was not making the appointments himself but sending requests or recommendations to men in the war department such as Simon Cameron, Lorenzo Thomas, or Edwin Stanton. One of the physicians Lincoln recommended was Isaac Israel Hayes, an Arctic explorer who wished to serve as a brigade surgeon. Lincoln wrote to Stanton that "I would like for him to be appointed at once, if consistent with the rules." Hayes received his commission and was in charge of the Satterlee Hospital in Philadelphia from May 1862 to June 1865. Even Vice President Hannibal Hamlin recommended his nephew for brigade surgeon, and Lincoln noted, "I hope he can be obliged."[10]

Although the Union army continued its practice of appointing regimental chaplains, initially there was no provision for hospital chaplains. A number of "Christian Ministers, and other pious people" brought this deficiency to Lincoln's attention. The president came to believe that "the services of chaplains are more needed, perhaps, in the hospitals, than with the healthy soldiers in the field." Lincoln did not think that he had the power to appoint such chaplains, but in October 1861 he suggested to several ministers that if they volunteered as hospital chaplains, he would ask Congress to pay them at the same rate as regimental chaplains. As promised, Lincoln included this explanation and request in his annual message of December 3, 1861.[11]

After Congress passed a law in the spring of 1862 that permitted Lincoln to appoint hospital chaplains, the president received many requests for appointments. Some came from regimental chaplains whose health had broken under the harsh field conditions but who believed that they could still serve the soldiers in a more protected environment. In one case, a chaplain from a disbanded regiment asked to serve in a hospital. Lincoln's friend Orville H. Browning requested the appointment of Mr. Emery as hospital chaplain at Quincy, Illinois, Browning's hometown. Even the Lincolns' pastor in Washington, Phineas D. Gurley, recommended Reverend Van Santvoord, a former regimental chaplain, for a Washington hospital post. Although it took some months, Lincoln finally asked Surgeon General Hammond to assign Van Santvoord to the convalescent camp.[12] Lincoln eventually had the opportunity to recommend medical inspectors also.[13]

Many people also called upon Lincoln to resolve problems of various sorts. Some needed exceptions to the rules, such as the extension of a leave of absence. Others resigned for health or other reasons and later wished to be reinstated. Several had been relieved from duty without explanation and sought to find the cause.[14]

Similarly, Lincoln's approval, disapproval, or intervention was often sought in various kinds of discipline cases. Medical officers who did not have military backgrounds and did not understand proper procedures often came into conflict with military officers, leading to many courts-martial. Surgeons were court-martialed for alleged drunkenness and for stealing two one-dollar bills from a drawer, for example. Sometimes the accusations indicated serious breaches of military discipline, but at times the charges proved to be petty retaliation by a surgeon's enemies. In other cases, what sounded like serious charges had feasible explanations. For instance, Dr. George W. New of the Seventh Indiana Infantry was accused of selling hospital whiskey to soldiers; however, he did this because there was no transportation to bring it along when the regiment moved. New had intended to use the proceeds for the purchase of medicinal whiskey at their new location. In another case, Surgeon Alfred Wynkoop was court-martialed for giving information to a Confederate sympathizer; however, he had done so unintentionally. Several of the surgeons charged with being absent without leave had encountered problems with their paperwork that were beyond their control. Lincoln carefully considered the cases brought before him, at times asking Judge Advocate General Joseph Holt or other appropriate persons for more information. In some cases, Lincoln approved the findings of the court. In other situations, he urged mitigation of the punishment, such as not dismissing the medical officer from the army.[15]

One of the most egregious cases Lincoln faced was that of Dr. David M. Wright. On July 11, 1863, in Norfolk, Virginia, Wright shot and killed Lieutenant Alanson L. Sanborn of Company B, First US Colored Troops, because Wright objected to Sanborn's drilling his black soldiers on the sidewalks of Main Street. A military commission found Wright guilty and sentenced him to death. Wright's lawyers tried to appeal with an insanity defense. Lincoln sent Dr. John P. Gray, an expert on sanity issues, to examine Wright. When the numerous reports and investigations declared Wright sane, Lincoln approved of the sentence that Wright be hanged and refused to countermand the order.[16]

In general, Lincoln was concerned about overly harsh punishments. He cautioned Stanton against "the dismissal of officers when neither incompetency, nor intentional wrong, nor real injury to the service is imputed. In such cases it is both cruel and impolitic, to crush the man, and make him and his friends permanent enemies to the administration if not to the government itself."[17]

At times Lincoln played a part in promoting medical products and services. Lincoln passed on to Surgeon General Hammond the recommendation of his family physician, Dr. Robert K. Stone, that the medical department use a disinfectant developed by a Dr. Kidwell. Lincoln also evidently forwarded the solicitation of Dr. S. W. Forsha, who had invented some sort of "balm" that would supposedly heal wounds. The president could, and did, testify from personal experience that Dr. Isachar Zacharie had successfully treated Lincoln's own foot problems and could be beneficial to the soldiers. In what was no doubt a change of pace, Lincoln inquired of Congress whether Surgeon Solomon Sharp of the Naval Hospital at Norfolk, Virginia, could accept a "piece of plate" (silverware) offered to Sharp in thanks from two British naval officers whom he had treated.[18]

Lincoln also aided women nurses in various ways. In some instances, he provided letters of introduction or tried to help women get to the areas where they wanted to serve. He issued a pass with "transportation to any of the Armies" for Annie Wittenmeyer, a relief worker from Iowa. Lincoln ordered a discharge from the army for the ailing youngest son of Abigail C. Berea, a volunteer nurse who had lost her husband and another son in the war. Cordelia Harvey, widow of the Wisconsin governor who had worked in several western hospitals herself, had a series of meetings with Lincoln over four days, probably in 1863. She eventually persuaded Lincoln about the importance of establishing hospitals in the North for long-term recuperation of the soldiers.[19]

A group of male nurses at the Columbian College Hospital in Washington petitioned Lincoln for assistance in getting paid. Most of them had been working for seven months and had received nothing but excuses, despite the provision of their contract that they were supposed to be paid monthly. Most of them had dependent families who were suffering hardship, and they applied to Lincoln because the nurses did not know where else to turn. The petition, referred by Lincoln to Stanton, itself got the runaround, ending with an endorsement by Surgeon General Hammond that suggests that the nurses may have suffered as part of Stanton's vendetta against Hammond.[20]

Rebecca Pomroy, who nursed Tad Lincoln through typhoid fever and Mary Lincoln after a carriage accident, was a special case in the Lincolns' lives. In March 1862, as Tad and Mary were convalescing, Pomroy spent some days at the hospital and some at the White House. Lincoln took her back to the Columbian College Hospital, where she normally worked, in the White House carriage. Lincoln and Mary sent along flowers from the White House conservatory, pictures, potted plants, and fruit for the soldiers. In turn, when Pomroy had malaria and needed a rest furlough, which her supervisor Dorothea Dix would not grant, Lincoln requested that Pomroy be stationed at the White House for several weeks to be with Mary because Mary's sister Elizabeth Edwards had been called home. Pomroy apparently spent three weeks at the White House. She encouraged both Mary and Lincoln to visit the hospitalized soldiers. Pomroy recounted one visit that Lincoln made to the Columbian College Hospital with Orville H. Browning. As she gave a tour through the buildings and tents, Lincoln shook the hand of each soldier, asking his name and regiment. At Christmas 1862, Mary sent flowers and two barrels of apples to the patients at Pomroy's hospital. Pomroy also had several getaway visits at the White House in the spring of 1863. In gratitude to Pomroy personally, whom he called "one of the best women I ever knew," Lincoln requested that Stanton appoint George K. Pomroy, her only surviving child, a second lieutenant in the regular US Army, which Stanton did.[21]

Although the Lincolns had a special relationship with Pomroy and the Columbian College Hospital, they did not restrict their attention to the soldiers of that facility. It is not possible to say how often Lincoln visited hospitals, but enough accounts exist to show that he went frequently. Certainly he sometimes visited in the aftermath of particular battles. Shortly after First Manassas (Bull Run), Lincoln and

Secretary of State William H. Seward visited the General Hospital in Georgetown on July 31 and August 3, 1861. In October 1862, after the Battle of Antietam, Lincoln went to that field to visit General George B. McClellan and the Army of the Potomac. They also stopped to see General Israel B. Richardson, who had been seriously wounded. Then Lincoln visited a barn full of Confederate wounded, to whom he spoke kindly and with whom he shook hands. On Christmas Day 1862, Lincoln and Mary called at a number of Washington hospitals. Lincoln is also known to have visited hospitals of the Army of the Potomac at Falmouth, Virginia, in April 1863 and at City Point, Virginia, in April 1865, on which occasion he shook more than 5,000 hands. With Senator James Doolittle of Wisconsin, Lincoln stopped at three Washington hospitals on May 24, 1863, shaking more than 1,000 hands. Lincoln and Mary spent time at Columbian College Hospital on May 13, 1864, and at Campbell Hospital on May 29, where they comforted a soldier who had just had his leg amputated. On another occasion, Lincoln witnessed an amputation at the shoulder joint, a risky operation at the time.[22]

It is important to realize that Lincoln's hospital visits were not the Civil War equivalent of a photo opportunity where the president breezed in, shook a few carefully cleaned hands, and made sure journalists saw that he "cared" about the health of the soldiers. Those who reported on these visits noted that Lincoln shook the hands of everyone able to do so in the ward or the hospital and spoke encouragingly to them. He took a great deal of time with the patients as a group, even though he could spend little with each individual.

Although Mary visited hospitals with Lincoln, she also frequently went by herself or with friends, such as Mary Jane Welles, bringing flowers and delicacies. When Mary received a donation of $1,000 for hospital relief work in August 1862, she ordered $200 worth of lemons and $100 worth of oranges for the patients. In early October, Mary sent 1,000 pounds of grapes to the hospitals. Mrs. Caleb B. Smith, wife of the secretary of the interior, evidently coordinated efforts to provide Christmas dinner for the hospitalized soldiers in 1862. Mary furnished a great deal of food for the occasion. Sometimes Tad went with Mary. At least once, in August 1864, Mary wrote a letter to a woman for her disabled son in the Campbell Hospital. Even Robert Lincoln visited a hospital on occasion, conversing with and translating for a Frenchman in the Columbian College Hospital.[23]

In addition to visiting hospitals, Lincoln was called upon to assist with hospitals and medically related buildings in other ways. He granted Illinois governor Richard Yates permission to use government land in Springfield, Illinois, to erect a soldiers' home to minister to soldiers in transit to and from their regiments. On some occasions, Lincoln talked with people about establishing hospitals in several places. He also at times intervened in one way or another when people complained about buildings being occupied for medical purposes. In one case, he ordered the return of a schoolhouse to its normal functions rather than permitting it to continue to be used for the Army Medical Museum.[24]

Lincoln also received requests to attend to the needs of many individual soldiers. Some of the requests were especially related to the soldiers' mental or physical health. When Private Lorenzo C. Stewart of the Fourteenth New York Artillery accidentally murdered two guards with morphine while trying to escape from jail, Lincoln ordered an examination of the man's sanity and ultimately commuted his death sentence to ten years at hard labor. Some soldiers were sentenced to be shot for desertion or punished for other infractions, but relatives or friends presented questions about the soldiers' sanity. In some cases, Lincoln ordered further investigation; in others, he modified the punishment or discharged the soldier from the army.[25]

Some parents wrote to Lincoln requesting him to discharge their underage sons who had enlisted without permission and were now sick. Lincoln ordered physical examinations and discharges for many other soldiers whose illnesses prevented their effective service.[26] The president even paroled or discharged some Confederate prisoners of war who were seriously ill and whose relatives requested their release.[27] He also ordered investigations of injustices done to sick and wounded soldiers, such as dismissal from the service, because of misunderstandings during their convalescence. In addition, Lincoln supported the efforts of some disabled soldiers to find non-military or less taxing jobs.[28]

Lincoln clearly favored the payment of pensions to disabled sol-diers, as well as to "the widows, orphans, and dependent mothers of those who have fallen in battle, or died of disease contracted, or of wounds received in the service of their country." As he reported in his fourth annual message on December 6, 1864, 16,770 disabled soldiers and 271 seamen had been added to the pension rolls between July 1, 1863, and June 30, 1864. In that same period, $4,504,616.92 had been paid to pensioners of all types (including beneficiaries from the Revolutionary War).[29]

Lincoln also, on occasion, paid attention to medical situations affecting generals and other officials. Perhaps the most important instance was General George B. McClellan's bout with typhoid fe-ver from December 23, 1861, into mid-January 1862. Lincoln visited McClellan on business but also sought to shield the general from an-noyances such as military decision-making and brass bands that were disturbing McClellan's rest. Much to the general's dismay, Lincoln began to exert more leadership in military matters and never fully relinquished it, even after McClellan recovered.[30]

When other military officers were wounded, Lincoln visited them if possible. He saw Lieutenant John L. Worden, commander of the ironclad *Monitor*, whose vision had been damaged during the ves-sel's battle with the *Merrimac*. Lincoln and Tad went to visit Daniel E. Sickles when that general arrived in Washington just after the Battle of Gettysburg, where Sickles had been wounded and had his leg amputated. Although Lincoln could not visit his friend General Richard J. Oglesby, who had been wounded at the Battle of Corinth, Mississippi, on October 3, 1862, he inquired after Oglesby's health. In several instances, Lincoln awarded promotions to dying officers, as a last sign of respect for their sacrifice.[31]

Lincoln's concern for the sick was not restricted to the military. Congressman Owen Lovejoy, with whom Lincoln had been acquaint-ed in Illinois and who supported Lincoln as president, was in declining health for some months before his death on March 25, 1864. Lincoln visited Lovejoy frequently during the congressman's illness. The presi-dent also made provisions to take care of William Johnson's paycheck and burial expenses when Johnson, his valet, sickened and died from smallpox. On April 5, 1865, while Lincoln was at City Point, Secretary of State Seward was seriously injured in a carriage accident. One of the first things Lincoln did upon his return to Washington was to visit Seward. After Lewis Payne wounded Seward on April 14 as part of the assassination conspiracy, no one told Seward that Lincoln was dead. However, Seward guessed it himself because Lincoln had not come to see him or at least inquired about his health.[32]

The Sanitary Commission and its affiliate organizations raised and spent a great deal of money to provide supplies and care for sick and wounded soldiers during the war. One of the major fund-raising activities for the commission during the latter half of the war was the "sanitary fair." Devised by a group of women in Chicago, over the protests of their male colleagues who did not think the women would be able to manage such an enterprise, the first fair was held October 27–November 7, 1863, and was widely imitated thereafter. At least thirty were held nationwide, but only Chicago staged a second one, in 1865. In most cases, the fairs were primarily planned, managed, and staffed by women of all ages who invited the general public to attend the fund-raiser. These fairs charged admission and included extensive exhibits of artifacts, collections, homemade products, and artwork, most of which was donated and for sale. Women staffed booths selling food of many kinds. The fairs also featured raffles, contests, parades, dances, concerts, and other entertainment. Notable people were invited to contribute items for sale to the highest bidder. Lincoln was no exception in this regard. In fact, he sent his original draft of the Emancipation Proclamation to the Chicago fair. The purchaser, Thomas Barbour Bryan, paid $3,000 and had lithographic copies made that were also sold for the benefit of the Sanitary Commission. Lincoln even won the gold pocket watch that had been offered as an incentive to the person who made the largest contribution to the fair.[33]

The sponsors of many other fairs also contacted Lincoln, and he contributed to them as well. He donated a copy of his Amnesty Proclamation of December 8, 1863, to the Great Western Fair in Cincinnati held later that December. Because the original document was in poor condition, Lincoln recopied the entire piece, with the same alterations he had made in the original. The framed document sold for $150. Lincoln was unable to attend the Sailor's Fair in Boston in November 1864, but on November 8, Lincoln was presented with a "mammoth Ox" named General Grant with the idea that he, in turn, would present it to the fair to be sold for the benefit of the sailors. The sale of the ox netted $3,200 for the fair. Lincoln also sat for a bust that appeared at the Great Central Sanitary Fair in Philadelphia. The original draft of the preliminary Emancipation Proclamation went to the Albany, New York, Army Relief Bazaar in Aid of the Sanitary Commission (February 22–March 5, 1864). Here the committee sold 1,100 chances on the document for one dollar each. Fittingly, the winner was the abolitionist Gerrit Smith, who donated the document to the Sanitary Commission. In 1865, the commission sold the proclamation to the New York legislature for $1,000. Edward Everett donated a copy of his Gettysburg speech, bound with a copy of Lincoln's in the president's own hand, to be sold at the New York City fair.[34]

Lincoln sent a number of more ordinary autograph letters to fairs such as those in Brooklyn, Philadelphia, and St. Louis. Not all of Lincoln's donations sold well, however. Notes that Lincoln had used for a speech on March 5, 1860, in Hartford, Connecticut, did not sell at the New York City fair and were sent on to the Philadelphia fair in June 1864. The Philadelphia fair attempted to sell fifty copies of a broadside of the Emancipation Proclamation signed by Lincoln and Secretary of State Seward with an attestation by John Nicolay. Only a few sold, and five of the remainder were sent on to the Sailor's Fair in Boston in November 1864.[35]

It was easier for Lincoln to comply with requests for autographs than to accept invitations to attend the fairs. He sent congratulatory messages and encouragement to the organizers, but most of the fairs were beyond the distance Lincoln thought wise to travel outside Washington.[36] Lincoln did, however, attend three fairs, in Washington, Baltimore, and Philadelphia.

The Washington fair was held in the patent office building and opened on February 22, 1864. Lincoln, Mary, Robert, and Lincoln's friend Richard J. Oglesby were among those who attended the exercises that evening. After a speech by Lucius E. Chittenden and a poem by Benjamin B. French, the audience called for Lincoln to speak. As the committee that invited Lincoln to the fair had not asked him to speak, he had not prepared to do so. Lincoln talked extemporaneously and humorously for several minutes about why he was not going to give a speech. On the way home, Mary berated Lincoln for giving the worst speech she had ever heard, which completely mortified her. Lincoln attended the fair again on the night it closed. This time his speech commended not only the sacrifice of the soldiers but also the work of the women who put together the fairs to raise funds for soldier relief.[37]

Lincoln traveled to Baltimore to address the opening of its fair on the evening of April 18, 1864. His speech actually had little to do with the fair itself as Lincoln talked about varying definitions of liberty and the possibility that there had been a massacre at Fort Pillow. Gideon Welles noted Lincoln's support for the fairs, commenting in his diary that Lincoln missed the cabinet meeting on April 19 because the president had been at the Baltimore fair with Postmaster General Montgomery Blair, a Maryland resident. Welles remarked that Lincoln "has a fondness for attending these shows only surpassed by Seward."[38]

The most physically demanding of Lincoln's visits was to the Great Central Sanitary Fair in Philadelphia. Initially, Lincoln was invited to speak at the opening of the fair on June 7, 1864. He declined, probably because the 1864 Union (Republican) Party nominating convention was beginning in Baltimore at the same time and the president needed to pay attention to reports from that gathering. He recommended Methodist bishop Matthew Simpson for his replacement speaker. Once Lincoln was safely renominated, he did visit the fair with Mary and Tad. The party left Washington by train at 7:00 A.M. on June 16, arriving about 11:30 A.M. and proceeding to the Continental Hotel. After lunch, the group went to the fairgrounds around 4:00. Everywhere Lincoln went, it was extremely crowded. It was difficult for Lincoln to move from place to place or to see any of the exhibits. The fact that the admission price was doubled

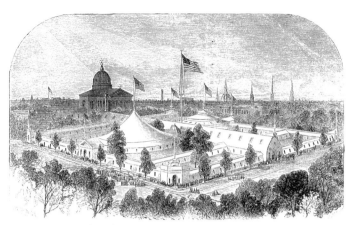

GREAT CENTRAL FAIR BUILDINGS,
Logan Square, Philadelphia, June, 1864.

Layout of the Great Central Sanitary Fair, Philadelphia, June 7–28, 1864. Union Avenue is the arched structure running from left to right through the grounds. The circular building on its left is the horticultural or floral department. On the right, the shorter circular building is a restaurant. The sanitary fair in Philadelphia was one of the largest in the country, raising $1,035,398.96 for the United States Sanitary Commission, second only to the amount raised in New York City in April 1864. *Our Daily Fare*, June 20, 1864, after 94; Abraham Lincoln Presidential Library and Museum (ALPLM).

(from fifty cents to one dollar per person) on the day of Lincoln's visit simply raised more money rather than restricted attendance. At a 7:00 P.M. banquet, Lincoln made a brief speech commending the motives of this and other fairs and discussing what might be needed to end the war. He went on to a reception at the Union League Club and spoke briefly from the balcony at his hotel about midnight. In both cases, his speech consisted mainly of explaining that he came to Philadelphia to support the fair. Lincoln returned to Washington on June 17 while Mary and Tad went on to New York.[39]

As part of the responsibilities of his presidency, Lincoln became involved with medical issues more generally, beyond his personal and family requirements. Throughout the war, he had a tendency

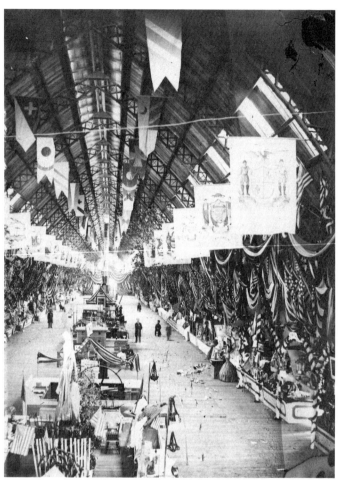

Union Avenue at the Great Central Sanitary Fair. Union Avenue, the central hall of the fair, was 540 feet long and 64 feet wide under 50-foot-tall Gothic arches. It contained decorations and exhibits throughout and was the architectural centerpiece of the fair. The original photo is faded. When Abraham Lincoln attended the fair with Mary and Tad on June 16, Union Avenue was so crowded with people that the president could hardly see the exhibits. Charles J. Stillé, *Memorial of the Great Central Fair for the U.S. Sanitary Commission* (Philadelphia: United States Sanitary Commission, 1865), between 32 and 33; Abraham Lincoln Presidential Library and Museum (ALPLM).

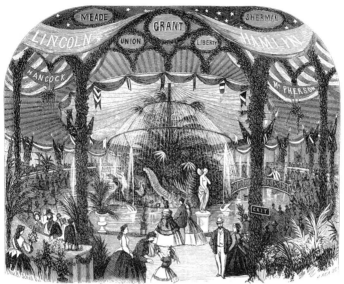

THE FLORAL DEPARTMENT OF THE GREAT CENTRAL FAIR.

The floral department of the Great Central Sanitary Fair. Housed in a circular structure 190 feet in diameter, partly covered with canvas, the department included a fountain, a lake, lights, and many ornamental plants. It was considered one of the highlights of the sanitary fair. *Our Daily Fare*, June 20, 1864, 93; Abraham Lincoln Presidential Library and Museum (ALPLM).

to delegate and defer to his cabinet members and military leaders as those who should know most about the needs of their own departments, unless, or until, they proved their incompetence. This is a sensible method of leadership. The emphasis of the war department was always on recruiting, training, and supplying troops. Medical care occupied a subordinate place for the army and, consequently, for Lincoln, who deferred to Stanton more than twenty-first-century readers might wish. As Lincoln told Benjamin French, "I can over rule his decision if I will, but I cannot well administer the War Department independent of the Secretary of War."[40]

THE ASSASSINATION OF LINCOLN

T he theater had been a means of relaxation and escape for Abraham Lincoln throughout the Civil War. When he and Mary went to see the silly play *Our American Cousin* at Ford's Theatre one April evening, they did not expect anything different. Tragically, the night of April 14, 1865, was very different indeed.

Shortly after 10:00 P.M., Southern-sympathizing actor John Wilkes Booth entered the presidential box and shot Lincoln in the back of the head at point-blank range before jumping to the stage and making his escape. As the audience came to realize that this was not a part of the play, chaos ensued. When someone called frantically for a doctor, the first to respond was Charles A. Leale, who was seated in the dress circle about forty feet from Lincoln's box.

It might not have inspired much confidence if people had realized that Leale was twenty-three and had received his medical degree from Bellevue Hospital Medical College in New York only six weeks earlier. In fact, that very day, April 14, Leale had been promoted from acting assistant surgeon to the commissioned post of assistant surgeon, to date from April 8. He was in charge of a wounded officers' ward at the Armory Square Hospital in Washington. However, despite his recent acquisition of credentials, Leale had had a great deal of appropriate experience during the war. He had studied gunshot wounds and surgery privately with the noted Dr. Frank H. Hamilton. Leale had also been part of the Union army's medical cadet program from February 17, 1864, to February 17, 1865. This involved a year of very practical training, experience, and increasing responsibility, most likely for Leale in a ward of the Armory Square Hospital. As a result, Leale was an appropriate person to care for the wounded president.[1]

Leale left two accounts of his treatment of Lincoln: a letter written to Benjamin F. Butler on July 21, 1867, for the House Special Committee on Lincoln's Assassination, and a recollection, *Lincoln's Last Hours*, printed after it was delivered as a talk to the New York Commandery of the Military Order of the Loyal Legion of the United States in honor of Lincoln's one hundredth birthday in 1909. Both of these accounts were based on notes written soon after the event. Many of Leale's memories are confirmed in the journal and memoir of Dr. Charles Sabin Taft, who arrived at the presidential box in Ford's Theatre shortly after Leale.[2]

When Leale entered the box, he found Lincoln with his eyes closed and his head leaning to the right, being held upright in his chair by the weeping Mary. In all the confusion, Leale could feel no pulse and realized Lincoln was "almost dead." "His breathing was exceedingly stertorious [harsh snoring and gasping], there being intervals between each inspiration and he was in a most profoundly comatozed condition." Two men helped Leale lay Lincoln on the floor. Noticing some blood near Lincoln's left shoulder, Leale remembered seeing Booth's knife and initially looked without success for an arterial stab wound. When Leale lifted Lincoln's eyelids, he saw that the pupil of one eye was dilated, a sign of brain injury. Feeling through Lincoln's hair, Leale found the gunshot wound "in the back part of the head, behind the left ear." A blood clot with matted hair blocked the opening. Leale removed this with his fingers, gently probing the wound with his little finger. As the wound began to bleed a bit, Lincoln's vital signs improved. Leale and the other doctors had to periodically remove blood clots throughout the night, relieving the pressure on his brain, to keep Lincoln alive.[3]

Some people have suggested that because the doctors probed Lincoln's wound with their fingers, infection was introduced and was the cause of Lincoln's death. While it is no question that wound infections were a cause of serious illness and death during the war, this was not the problem in Lincoln's case. Had Leale *not* poked around in Lincoln's wound, the president would have died within a few minutes on the floor of the theater box. Probing the wound and removing blood clots actually kept Lincoln alive for about nine more hours.[4]

Leale also gave Lincoln a type of artificial respiration. While two assistants moved Lincoln's arms up and down, Leale pressed his diaphragm upward, helping Lincoln to breathe, while also performing a bit of external heart massage. Several times Leale also provided a type of mouth-to-mouth breathing. With Lincoln temporarily stable, Leale answered the question of the president's prognosis: "His wound is mortal; it is impossible for him to recover."[5] Despite this diagnosis, Leale and the other doctors did all they could to keep Lincoln alive as long as possible.

After giving Lincoln a tiny bit of brandy and water as a stimulant, Leale determined that the president should be moved from the theater. Leale believed that Lincoln would die on the way if he were taken to the White House, a decision supported by Drs. Taft and Albert F. A. King, who were then assisting him. The three doctors and some other men carefully carried Lincoln to the Peterson house across the street. In the back bedroom, Lincoln was placed diagonally on the bed because he was too tall for it and the footboard could not be removed. All of this took no more than twenty minutes.[6]

Once Lincoln was situated, Leale and the other doctors examined the president to see if he had any other wounds, which he did not. To warm Lincoln's cold feet and legs, Leale ordered hot water bottles and hot blankets to be applied, as well as a mustard plaster all over Lincoln's front. Leale also, as necessary, removed blood clots from the wound to relieve brain pressure. However, he administered no medicines of any kind. Taft and King alternated in keeping Lincoln's head comfortably on the pillow.[7]

Leale also sent for Lincoln's son Robert; the Lincoln family physician, Robert K. Stone; Leale's superior at the Armory Square Hospital, D. Willard Bliss; Surgeon General Joseph K. Barnes and Assistant Surgeon General Charles H. Crane; the Lincolns' pastor, Phineas D. Gurley; and all the cabinet members. As the ranking physicians arrived, Leale explained the wound, his diagnosis, and his treatment.

Each doctor approved and continued the same procedures until the president's death.[8]

Surgeon General Barnes and Leale explored the wound with a Nelaton probe, a long, thin rod with a white porcelain bulb on the tip. If the porcelain touched the bullet, the lead projectile would leave a mark on the porcelain. In the days before X-rays, a probe could help doctors determine where a bullet was, if it could be removed or not (some soldiers lived with a bullet for decades), and if there was other foreign matter in the wound. In Lincoln's case, the doctors apparently found loose bone pieces after several inches and may have touched the bullet as far as seven inches into the brain. No further explorations were made. The doctors simply continued comfort measures.[9]

After the other doctors took charge, Leale remained with Lincoln, holding his right hand and occasionally checking his pulse. Although he assumed that Lincoln was blind and paralyzed, Leale also realized that in his coma Lincoln might still be able to hear or feel, so he wanted Lincoln to have the comfort of human contact. Near dawn on April 15, it was clear to all that Lincoln was "sinking." His pulse became infrequent, with his breathing sporadic and "guttural." Lincoln died at 7:22 in the morning.[10]

Although no one's treatment could have saved Lincoln, Leale believed that his efforts in keeping Lincoln alive for nine more hours were beneficial. On a purely personal level, Robert Lincoln got to see his father still alive. Lincoln's lingering also furthered the security of the country, giving time for governmental leaders to assemble and prepare for the transition, to gather the military, and to calm crowds of people.[11]

After Lincoln's body was transported to the White House, an autopsy was conducted only of Lincoln's head. Some modern doctors have lamented that had a full autopsy been performed, information concerning Lincoln's heart could have answered questions about whether he had such diseases as syphilis or Marfan syndrome. However, in 1865, doing any autopsy at all was fairly uncommon, and the doctors were interested only in the nature of Lincoln's wound. At 11:00 A.M., Joseph J. Woodward, a noted surgeon and medical historian, and Dr. Edward Curtis (whose bloodstained shirt cuffs that he wore that day are at the National Museum of Health and Medicine in Washington, DC) performed the procedure. Surgeon General Barnes; Assistant Surgeon General Crane; Drs. Taft, Stone, and William Notson; General Christopher C. Augur; and new president Andrew Johnson attended the autopsy. Leale was invited but declined because he believed his patients at the Armory Square Hospital required his services.[12]

In addition to Woodward's autopsy report, Taft also left a rather detailed account of the autopsy procedure and what the doctors found. Essentially, the bullet pierced Lincoln's skull about an inch to the left of the middle of his head, taking some bone fragments into the wound. The bullet crossed the brain at a slight angle, but the accounts disagree about whether it stopped behind Lincoln's left eye (Woodward and Stone) or right eye (Barnes and Taft). Since Secretary of the Navy Gideon Welles noted in his diary that about an hour after he was shot, Lincoln's right eye began to swell and that side of his face began to discolor, the right may well be the correct side. At any rate, the doctors performing the autopsy removed and examined Lincoln's brain. They also discovered that the bones of his eye sockets had been fractured. Blood had congealed in various parts of the brain, while other areas, including the brainstem, which controls breathing and automatic functions, were not affected.[13]

One thing that clearly impressed the doctors was Lincoln's physique. Dr. Curtis reported to his mother a few days after the autopsy that "I was simply astonished at the showing of the nude remains, where well-founded muscles built on strong bones, told the powerful athlete. Now I understand the prowess recorded in the President's early days." Even Gideon Welles, while visiting the dying Lincoln, noted, "His large arms, which were occasionally exposed, were of a size which one would scarce have expected from his spare appearance."[14] It should be noted that whatever ailments may have affected Lincoln during the last months of his life and whatever caused his face to age did not diminish the muscular strength of his body.

After the autopsy, Stone and Taft took the bullet, the bone fragments, and the Nelaton probe to Secretary of War Edwin M. Stanton, who sealed them in envelopes. These artifacts are presently part of the

National Museum of Health and Medicine collection. Dr. Charles D. Brown, of the undertaking firm Brown and Alexander, embalmed Lincoln's body, preparing it as well as possible for the more than 1,600-mile cross-country train journey and twelve funerals. Lincoln's body was finally deposited in a temporary receiving vault at Oak Ridge Cemetery in Springfield, Illinois, on May 4, 1865.[15]

Periodically, people wonder whether Lincoln could actually have survived the assassination, especially if it had occurred in a later century with more treatment options. According to Leale, he had never seen or heard of a person with a similar wound who had survived or even lived for an hour. At the time, others also expressed surprise that Lincoln had survived nine hours. In May 1960, Lieutenant Colonel George J. Hayes, chief of neurological service at Walter Reed Army Hospital, said that with the best treatment available in 1960, Lincoln would have had at most a 50–50 chance of survival. Survival, of course, would not mean complete recovery. Hayes speculated that Lincoln would have been "completely paralyzed on the right side and possibly unable to talk."[16] Only three years later, President John F. Kennedy did not survive a similar gunshot wound.

In 2007, Thomas M. Scalea, director of the Shock Trauma Center in Baltimore, addressed the Thirteenth Historical Clinicopathological Conference on the topic. In the twenty-first century, there would be far more hope for Lincoln's survival because critical parts of the brain, such as the brainstem, were not damaged. Treatment methods could include temporarily removing part of the skull to relieve pressure and remove pooled blood; standing the bed on the foot end to relieve pressure; replacing lost fluids and giving medications intravenously; and perhaps other procedures. Again, however, the result would be limited. "If he had lived, he would at the very least have been partially blind, unsteady on his feet, numb in certain regions of his body and inarticulate. Nevertheless, he might have been able to think and, after much rehabilitation, communicate."[17]

Ultimately, then, in no scenario so far possible could Lincoln have recovered from his wound sufficiently to remain an effective president. Once Booth fired his shot, Andrew Johnson was president.

CHAPTER SEVEN

LINCOLN'S FAMILY AFTER THE WAR

As Abraham Lincoln lay dying in the back bedroom of the Peterson house on the night of April 14–15, 1865, Mary frequently came in to see her husband. At one point, as she was sitting on a chair next to the bed, Lincoln's "breathing became very stertorous and the loud, unnatural noise frightened her in her exhausted, agonized condition. She sprang up suddenly with a piercing cry and fell fainting to the floor." Secretary of War Edwin M. Stanton entered the room and ordered Mary taken out and kept out. She never saw Lincoln alive again.[1]

With Lincoln's death, Mary took to her bed for some weeks of uncontrolled mourning. Elizabeth Keckly described one such "paroxysm of grief": "the wails of a broken heart, the unearthly shrieks, the terrible convulsions, the wild, tempestuous outbursts of grief from the soul." Keckly responded by applying cold water to Mary's head and being as soothing as possible. It is hardly surprising that Mary broke down emotionally after Lincoln's death. To have her husband shot right next to her was certainly traumatic. Yet Mary could think only of her own loss, rarely of anyone else's. Her hysteria frightened and upset Tad, who had lost not only his father but his chief playmate since the death of Willie and the banishment of the Taft brothers. Mary remained in isolation at the White House, weeks after courtesy should have made her vacate for Andrew Johnson and his family. She did not leave Washington until May 22.[2]

Not surprisingly, Mary had a severe headache on the way to Chicago, where she was moving. Once she arrived in the city, Mary continued to have headaches and indispositions at frequent intervals, probably even more often than indicated in her correspondence. As she moaned to Dr. Anson G. Henry in a letter of July 17, "If it were not for dear little Taddie, I would pray to die, I am so miserable. I still remain closeted in my rooms, take an occasional walk, in the park & as usual see no one." At the end of December, Mary reported to Mary Jane Welles that she was disabled by headaches about three days a week.[3] As Mary's post–Civil War letters show, she never considered herself a healthy woman and generally conveyed her latest health issues to her friends and acquaintances in her correspondence. Nicely summarized by historian Jason Emerson, Mary's "severe indispositions" included "weak nerves, migraines, chills, boils, joint pains, incontinence, swelling, insomnia, melancholia, and fatigue."[4]

After the Civil War, Tad, who had been largely undisciplined and uneducated, finally began to mature. Now age twelve, he was "growing very fast" during the summer of 1865. On October 10, Mary reported to the Lincoln boys' former tutor that Tad "goes to school & can almost read," certainly delayed development for a twelve-year-old. In mid-December, Tad had a very bad cold, nearly croup.[5]

By January 17, 1868, Robert had "put Tad into a very good school where he appears to be learning very fast." Mary had taken Tad to a dentist in Chicago, who believed Tad's "teeth should be gradually forced into a proper position by means of a spring frame set in his mouth." However, this type of orthodontia bothered Tad very much and made his speech less clear than usual. Robert was very concerned about Tad developing even more bad speech habits. After consulting another dentist, Robert had Tad stop wearing the dental appliance and took him instead to an elocution teacher named McCoy "to make him pronounce correctly." Apparently, this early type of speech therapy did begin to help.[6]

On October 1, 1868, just after Robert married Mary Eunice Harlan, Mary and Tad Lincoln left for Europe, where they spent the next several years. For a while they lived in Frankfurt am Main in Germany, where Tad attended a boarding school and Mary lived in a boardinghouse. When Mary got sick and could not afford a nurse, Tad would have to leave school to take care of her. Mary and Tad then spent time in England as a result of the upheaval caused by the Franco-Prussian War. In England and Germany, both Lincolns seem to have developed frequent upper respiratory infections. At times, the doctors sent Mary to Italy for her health, but Tad always stayed in school. By May 1871, when the Lincolns returned to the United States, Tad, at eighteen, had grown into a well-behaved young man who was very attentive to his mother.[7]

Tad apparently caught yet another cold on the voyage back to America, and this one he was unable to shake. He was quite ill by the time he and his mother arrived in Chicago. On June 8, Mary reported that Tad "has been *very* dangerously ill" and she had been up with him for ten nights. Under the care of three physicians, Tad at last was seeming to improve. Dr. N. S. Davis, the lung specialist, had told Mary "that *thus far*, his lungs are *not at all* diseased although water has been formed on part of his left lung, which is gradually decreasing." Tad had such trouble breathing that he had to sleep sitting up in a chair. One night he rose from his chair and fainted, apparently either causing or caused by a relapse. Although Tad occasionally showed signs of improvement, these were only temporary and were followed by further decline. After great and patient suffering, Tad Lincoln died about 7:30 on the morning of Saturday, July 15, 1871, of what the obituary called "dropsy of the chest," which caused "compression of the heart." Tad was buried with his father and two brothers at Oak Ridge Cemetery in Springfield in a temporary vault until the completion of the Lincoln tomb.[8]

There has been some debate among historians and doctors about the cause of Tad's death. However, by the 1950s, most interested people believed that "dropsy of the chest" probably was what is known as pleurisy. The fluid accumulation was not *in* Tad's lungs but in the pleural sacs around both lungs. Scholar Milton Shutes agreed with the suggestion of W. A. Evans that Tad's history of upper respiratory illnesses over the previous months, leading to fatal pleurisy, could have been provoked by tuberculosis.[9] Several of those who advocate the idea that Lincoln and some of his sons had Marfan syndrome have claimed that Tad's symptoms indicate that he died from congestive heart failure, a consequence of Marfan syndrome.

However, Gabor S. Boritt and Adam Borit, in their thorough study, disagreed with the Marfan syndrome theory and believed that Tad probably died from tuberculosis. Not surprisingly, John Sotos, who attributed the majority of Abraham Lincoln's health problems to MEN2B, claimed that Tad had MEN2B-related lip lumps instead of a possible partially cleft palate. Rather than having tuberculosis or pleurisy, Tad could have had a chest cancer related to MEN2B, according to Sotos.[10] While historians cannot know for certain, a history of upper respiratory infections and several years of residence in cold, damp locations make pleurisy, possibly with a tubercular component, a very logical possibility.

After Tad's death, Mary fell apart. She had clung to Tad after Lincoln's assassination in ways that were probably unhealthy for both mother and son. As she wrote to a friend in October 1871, "I have been utterly prostrated—by my deep grief, that my health has completely given way. Latterly, I am suffering greatly with violent palpitation of the heart." During this period, Mary lived at times in Chicago but also traveled to Wisconsin, Canada, Boston, and elsewhere in search of health.[11]

In early 1875, Mary was in Florida with her nurse/companion. On March 12, she sent a telegram to Robert's law partner, concerned that Robert was ill. Although Robert and his family were all in good health, Mary could not be persuaded that Robert was not dying. She immediately boarded a train for Chicago. Because she was estranged from Robert's wife, Mary stayed at the Grand Pacific Hotel. As Mary's behavior became increasingly peculiar, Robert stayed at the hotel as well. Mary had a number of hallucinations and delusions including hearing voices, believing part of Chicago was on fire, and thinking that people were trying to poison her. She seemed agitated and restless much of the time, could not be left alone, and was fearful of many irrational things. She spent money recklessly, buying forty pairs of curtains, for example. Mary also carried $57,000 in cash and bonds on her person. After two months of this, Robert, the doctors he called in, and his advisors David Davis, Leonard Swett, and Mary's cousin John T. Stuart all considered Mary sick, as well as at risk personally. They believed intervention to be necessary.[12]

After a notorious legal case in the 1850s, Illinois was more cautious than most states at the time, requiring a trial before a person could be committed to an insane asylum. Doctors, hotel personnel, and Robert all testified at the trial on May 19, 1875, to Mary's bizarre behavior but evidently told only as much as was necessary for commitment, not as many details as could have been revealed. Mary spent late May to September 1875 at the Bellevue Place Sanitarium in Batavia, Illinois, a private institution where she had quiet, roomy, comfortable quarters, a personal attendant, and the freedom of beautifully landscaped grounds. She was not confined in a barred cell, nor were any of the other women patients. Mary's mental and physical state improved, but she rebelled against being institutionalized. With the aid of Chicago lawyers Myra and James Bradwell, Mary was released to the home of her sister Elizabeth Edwards in Springfield. In June 1876, the court declared Mary competent to manage her own affairs, although she did have Jacob Bunn, a Springfield banker, in charge of her assets.[13]

One of the most common questions raised when dealing with the subject of the Lincolns and medicine concerns Mary's sanity. Was she insane? Another question logically follows: Did Robert railroad her into an asylum to get her money, as Mary charged and several historians have agreed? The answer to the second question is easier than the first. Records show that Robert did not appropriate Mary's money. He managed her assets carefully while he controlled them, spent his own money for her care, and grieved at having to go through a trial and have her in an institution.[14]

The question of Mary's sanity is very complex. As seen earlier, she was very moody and self-centered throughout her life and grieved extremely at losses, beyond what was normal even for the Victorian era. She also tended to be very extreme in her attitudes toward money, varying from miserly penny-pinching to reckless extravagance on unnecessary, sometimes even useless, items that she then hoarded. One historian called her a "financial bulimic." Some of her contemporaries reported that she had a monomania about money.[15]

Opinion has varied about whether Mary was truly insane. As early as 1867, Robert wrote to his future wife that his mother was sane on all subjects except money. David Davis considered Mary to be "deranged" since Lincoln's death, and perhaps even before it. Orville H. Browning thought Mary "demented" for several years before her insanity trial. Mary's closest cousins, John T. Stuart and Elizabeth Grimsley Brown, both agreed that Mary was insane and should have a conservator for her property. Elizabeth Edwards believed, based on what Mary had told her, that Mary's problems were caused by a fever and too much chloral hydrate.[16]

Historian Jean Baker agreed with the idea that Mary had had too much chloral hydrate, and others have supposed Mary had some sort of addiction. In an undated letter, Mary complained to her doctor, Willis Danforth, about her "excessive wakefulness" and asked him to send her four "more powders" since she had already taken the five he had left for her. Chloral hydrate became popular in the 1860s precisely because it induced natural sleep without becoming addictive or having other side effects, if taken in moderation. Emerson suggested that Mary had no drug addiction because her physician, Dr. Danforth, was a homeopath who would prescribe only minute doses of any medicine. In addition, the Bellevue records never show that Mary was treated for any withdrawal symptoms. Historian Catherine Clinton, however, pointed out that chloral hydrate mixed with alcohol would produce a knockout drink with various symptoms, including confusion. Chloral hydrate has been an ingredient in "date rape" drugs of the modern era.[17] No one knows how much medication of any sort Mary was really taking. If she were mixing chloral hydrate and some alcohol-based patent medicine, she could have caused problems for herself that she did not have at other times.

Mary also allegedly attempted suicide on the day she was supposed to be taken to Bellevue. She eluded her guards and went to three different pharmacies trying to get laudanum. An alert clerk thwarted her plan, giving her only burnt sugar water rather than the opiate, which would have been fatal in the amount she drank. Jean Baker believed that this suicide attempt never happened and blamed the story on the machinations of Robert. Most of the other historians who deal with the episode accept the account, suggesting that it was a one-time act of desperation resulting from Mary's severe depression over the trial and her impending institutionalization.[18]

W. A. Evans, in his study of Mary Lincoln's personality, believed that Mary was emotionally, not mentally, insane and that her hallucinations were not caused by drugs but possibly by her practice of spiritualism. Baker diagnosed Mary as narcissistic, a "victim" who always needed attention. Mark E. Neely and R. Gerald McMurtry believed that Mary was insane in the spring of 1875, but they could not be sure about any other time. They thought the best proof of her insanity was that she realized her behavior needed an explanation and thus she tried to blame her difficulties on too much chloral hydrate. According to one psychiatrist, Mary was psychotic and schizophrenic, especially in 1875. James S. Brust, another psychiatrist, who teamed up with Jason Emerson in his analysis of Mary's insanity crisis, demonstrated that the problem in the spring of 1875 was merely the most full-blown episode of Mary's lifelong experience with manic-depression, now known as bipolar disorder.[19]

Was Mary Lincoln insane? It is clearly easier to speculate than to know for sure. Evidence shows that she had various psychological and physical problems throughout her life. It does seem, however, that the intensity and nature of her problems were more severe in the spring of 1875 than at any other time, and she was unable to resolve her difficulties without help.

Mary was mortified by all aspects of her trial, her institutionalization, and the publicity surrounding these events. Because she blamed Robert most bitterly for her ordeal, and for anything else she could think of, the two became estranged until 1881. In 1876, after the second sanity trial, Mary moved to Europe, mostly living in France and sometimes Italy. She sought water cures (usually unsuccessful) and other treatments but still suffered colds, boils, and other ailments. Her medical problems worsened after she fell off a stepladder or chair in December 1879 while adjusting a picture on the wall and injured her spine. Thereafter, she complained in her letters about "my poor broken back."[20]

Mary finally returned to the United States, arriving in New York on October 15, 1880. She consulted a noted orthopedic doctor, Lewis A. Sayre, who reported that she had "inflammation of the spine, kidney trouble," and "mental depression." Mary moved back to Springfield and lived with her sister Elizabeth Edwards, taking another trip to New York (October 1881–March 1882) to see Dr. Sayre and be treated by "electric baths." On January 1, 1882, Sayre and three other doctors examined Mary and produced an affidavit to present to Congress so that she could have her pension increased. The doctors found that "Mrs. Lincoln is suffering from chronic inflammation of the spinal cord, chronic disease of the kidneys, and commencing cataract of both eyes." They further elaborated that the spinal ailment was reducing her ability to walk at all and already had made her unable to walk down stairs. Mary also had "reflex paralysis of the iris of the eye, and the reduction of the sight to one-tenth," as well as a narrowed field of vision. The doctors saw no hope of improvement and believed that she would continue to need an attendant in the future, as she already did.[21]

Mary returned to Springfield in March 1882 and completely retreated into a darkened room, lit only by candlelight. She never went outside and spent her time rummaging through her more than sixty trunks of silks and other hoarded items. She died on July 16, 1882, evidently of a stroke, at the age of sixty-four. Mary was buried in Oak Ridge Cemetery with her husband and three sons.[22]

Although doctors and historians generally concede that Mary died of a stroke, there is some controversy about the nature of her final illness. A number speculate that Mary had untreated diabetes, which would account for many of her symptoms. In 1999, Norbert Hirschhorn and Robert G. Feldman published an article diagnosing Mary with tabes dorsalis or locomotor ataxia, a chronic and progressive spinal cord disease characterized by widespread body pains; problems with walking, especially in the dark and down stairs; narrowed vision and difficulties with the pupils failing to contract when exposed to light; urinary incontinence; and joint swelling. These symptoms do largely match with the diagnosis of the four doctors, as well as Mary's complaints in her correspondence. Tabes dorsalis can be caused by syphilis (which Hirschhorn and Feldman pretty much rule out in Mary's case) or untreated diabetes. The four physicians suggested that Mary could have developed her problems from her fall in 1879, but Hirschhorn and Feldman proposed tabes dorsalis as a *cause* of Mary's fall.[23]

Once again, doctors have focused on a single disease to account for a multitude of symptoms in a Lincoln family member. And again, at this late date, no one can be sure. However, in this case, researchers do have the doctors' report of January 1, 1882, as well as Mary's frequent complaints as testimony to the possibility of diabetes and tabes dorsalis.

With Mary's death, Robert became the last surviving member of Lincoln's immediate family. A successful lawyer in Chicago, he was secretary of war (1881–85) and minister to Great Britain (1889–93), as well as president of the Pullman Company (1897–1911). He suffered great stress after Tad's death and, under doctor's orders, went away for several weeks of recuperation. At the time of Mary's insanity episode and trial, Robert did what he felt was his duty in the best interest of his mother, fulfilling his role as head of the family and a Victorian gentleman.[24]

During his later years, Robert did not have especially good health. He evidently had eye trouble for many years before he admitted to it in 1894. After a friend died in 1906, Robert had a nervous breakdown. When he attended the dedication of Abraham Lincoln's statue in Hodgenville, Kentucky, on Memorial Day 1909, shortly after Lincoln's one hundredth birthday, Robert was overcome with emotion, heat exhaustion, and possibly a small stroke. Due to poor health, Robert resigned as president of the Pullman Company in May 1911. For the rest of his life, Robert continued to have episodes of ill health, including another nervous breakdown, digestive problems, and chronic eye inflammation. It is possible that he may also have been somewhat of a hypochondriac, like his mother, and used his health as an excuse to avoid events in which he did not want to participate. Robert died of a stroke in his sleep during the night of July 25–26, 1926, just six days before his eighty-third birthday. He was buried at Arlington Cemetery just over the river from Washington, DC, rather than at Oak Ridge Cemetery in Springfield with the rest of the Lincoln family.[25]

So, did Lincoln have Marfan syndrome? Probably not. Was Mary insane? Probably not, but she was certainly having some difficulties. What did Willie die from? Probably typhoid fever, perhaps complicated by pneumonia.

As this study shows, it can be extremely difficult to properly diagnose the physical problems that afflicted Lincoln and his family. The remaining evidence is almost always too fragmentary to provide a conclusive answer. Nevertheless, enough information survives to test theories, narrow the options, and suggest logical conclusions. More than two hundred years after Abraham Lincoln's birth, interest in nearly every aspect of his life continues unabated. Lincoln's medical life is no exception to the trend. In some instances, however, people seem more eager to attach Lincoln's name to a particular cause or syndrome than to analyze the (sometimes meager) available evidence dispassionately.

While students of his life may not know precisely what affected Lincoln in many cases, they do know that he had frequent and increasing health problems while he was president. Despite these personal difficulties, Lincoln managed to conduct the affairs of state during the Civil War in such a way that he continues to be regarded by most as America's greatest president.

NOTES

BIBLIOGRAPHY

INDEX

NOTES

1. Young Lincoln, 1809–42

1. Sarah Bush Johnston Lincoln interview, Wilson and Davis, *Herndon's Informants*, 108; Austin Gollaher's comments in Charles Friend to Herndon, March 19, 1866, ibid., 235.

2. Lincoln, "Autobiography Written for John L. Scripps," ca. June 1860, *Collected Works*, 4:62; Dennis F. Hanks interview, Wilson and Davis, *Herndon's Informants*, 42; Burlingame, *Abraham Lincoln*, 1:24; White, *A. Lincoln*, 28–29; Shutes, *Lincoln and the Doctors*, 6; Garrison, *Lincoln No One Knows*, 17–18.

3. Prokopowicz, *Did Lincoln Own Slaves?*, 17; Boritt and Borit, "Lincoln and the Marfan Syndrome," 220; Fishman and Da Silveira, "Lincoln's Craniofacial Microsomia," 1128; Sotos, *Physical Lincoln*, 91–93.

4. Lincoln, "Autobiography Written for John L. Scripps," ca. June 1860, *Collected Works*, 4:62–63; Shutes, *Lincoln and the Doctors*, 17–18.

5. White, *A. Lincoln*, 100; Baker, *Mary Todd Lincoln*, 267–68; Burlingame, *Abraham Lincoln*, 1:98–101; Wilson, *Honor's Voice*, 114–26; Simon, "Abraham Lincoln and Ann Rutledge"; B. Schwartz, "Ann Rutledge in American Memory"; Gannett, "'Overwhelming Evidence.'"

6. The accounts by all the people who mentioned Lincoln and Rutledge can be found in Wilson and Davis, *Herndon's Informants*: William G. Greene interview, 21; Benjamin F. Irwin to Herndon, August 27, 1866, 325; Mentor Graham to Herndon, May 29, 1865, 11; Isaac Cogdal interview, 441; Henry McHenry to Herndon, January 8, 1866, 155–56; Caleb Carman to Herndon, November 30, 1866, 430; Thompson Ware McNeely to Herndon, November 12 and 28, 1866, 397 and 424; John Hill to Herndon, June 6, 1865, 23; James Short to Herndon, July 7, 1865, 73; Hardin Bale interview, 13; Robert B. Rutledge to Herndon, ca. November 1, 1866, 383; clipping from *Menard Axis*, February 15, 1862, 25; and Elizabeth Abell to Herndon, February 15, 1867, 557.

7. Shenk, *Lincoln's Melancholy*, 18–20. From Wilson and Davis, *Herndon's Informants*: William G. Greene interview, 21; Elizabeth Abell to Herndon, February 15, 1867, 557; John Hill to Herndon, June 6, 1865, 23; Mentor Graham to Herndon, May 29, 1865, 11; Henry McHenry interview and McHenry to Herndon, January 8, 1866, 14 and 155–56; Isaac Cogdal interview, 441.

8. Shutes, *Lincoln and the Doctors*, 17–18.

9. Lincoln to John T. Stuart, January 23, 1841, *Collected Works*, 1:229.

10. Lincoln to Joshua F. Speed, March 27, 1842, ibid., 282; Elizabeth Todd

Edwards interview, Wilson and Davis, *Herndon's Informants*, 443–44; Helm, *True Story of Mary*, 86–90; Burlingame, *Oral History*, xvi; Clinton, *Mrs. Lincoln*, 50–51; Donald, *"We Are Lincoln Men,"* 44; Shenk, *Lincoln's Melancholy*, 44–52, 55–56; White, *A. Lincoln*, 110–12.

11. Joshua F. Speed interview and Speed to Herndon, September 17, 1866, Wilson and Davis, *Herndon's Informants*, 495 and 342; Orville H. Browning interview, Burlingame, *Oral History*, 1–2; Shutes, *Lincoln and the Doctors*, 26–28; Shenk, *Lincoln's Melancholy*, 51–52, 57–59, 62–63; James C. Conkling to Mercy Ann Levering, January 24, 1841, Conkling Family Papers, box 1, folder 1, ALPL.

12. Sotos, *Physical Lincoln*, 228; Chambrun, "Personal Recollections," 32; Robert L. Wilson to Herndon, February 10, 1866, Wilson and Davis, *Herndon's Informants*, 205; Ward Hill Lamon interview, Wilson and Davis, *Herndon's Informants*, 466; Orville H. Browning interview, Burlingame, *Oral History*, 1–3; Shutes, *Lincoln and the Doctors*, 33.

13. Shutes, *Lincoln and the Doctors*, 33–35, 40, 42; Evans, *Mrs. Abraham Lincoln*, 329–31; Shenk, *Lincoln's Melancholy*, 13–15.

14. Sotos, *Physical Lincoln*, 216–19. For more information, see the discussion of Sotos and MEN2B in chapter 4.

15. Shenk, *Lincoln's Melancholy*, 22, 98–99, 108–9, 156; Goodwin, *Team of Rivals*, xvii, 103.

16. Shenk, *Lincoln's Melancholy*, 113, 156; Goodwin, *Team of Rivals*, xvii, 49, 103; Orville H. Browning interview, Burlingame, *Oral History*, 3.

17. Lincoln to Mary Owens, December 13, 1838, *Collected Works*, 1:54–55; Lincoln to Mary Speed, ibid., 1:260–61; Sotos, *Physical Lincoln*, 57.

18. Prokopowicz, *Did Lincoln Own Slaves?*, 46; Donald, *"We Are Lincoln Men,"* 98–99.

19. Donald, *"We Are Lincoln Men,"* 98; Wilson, *Honor's Voice*, 127–29, 182–84; Sotos, *Physical Lincoln*, 104.

20. For example, Simon, "Abraham Lincoln and Ann Rutledge." Donald, *"We Are Lincoln Men,"* 98–99; Shenk, *Lincoln's Melancholy*, 60.

21. Donald, *"We Are Lincoln Men,"* 99; Hirschhorn, Feldman, and Greaves, "Abraham Lincoln's Blue Pills," 323.

22. Lincoln to Samuel D. Marshall, November 11, 1842, *Collected Works*, 1:305.

2. The Lincoln Family, 1843–60

1. Information on Mary Lincoln's early life can be found in any biography, including Baker, *Mary Todd Lincoln*; Clinton, *Mrs. Lincoln*; Helm, *True Story of Mary*; and Berry, *House of Abraham*.

2. Woodrow quoted in Helm, *True Story of Mary*, 31–32; Bach, "Was Mary Todd Lincoln Bipolar?"

3. Baker, *Mary Todd Lincoln*, 73; Berry, *House of Abraham*, 14; Lincoln to Mary, April 16, 1848, *Collected Works*, 1:466; Turner and Turner, *Mary Todd Lincoln*, 32.

4. See any of the biographies listed in note 1.

5. Lincoln to Joshua Speed, October 22, 1846, *Collected Works*, 1:391; Baker, *Mary Todd Lincoln*, 124.

6. Frances Wallace interview in Wilson and Davis, *Herndon's Informants*, 485; Randall, *Lincoln's Sons*, 26–27; Goff, *Robert Todd Lincoln*, 17.

7. Randall, *Lincoln's Sons*, 11, 26; Clinton, *Mrs. Lincoln*, 89; Goff, *Robert Todd Lincoln*, 17; Durham, "Lincoln's Sons," 69. Marfan syndrome is discussed in chapter 4.

8. Lincoln to Joshua Speed, October 22, 1846, *Collected Works*, 1:391; Mary to Lincoln, May 1848, Turner and Turner, *Mary Todd Lincoln*, 37; Mary to Henry C. Deming, December 16, 1867, Schwartz and Bauer, "Unpublished Mary Todd Lincoln," 13–14; Lincoln to John D. Johnston, February 23, 1850, *Collected Works*, 2:76–77; "Edward Baker Lincoln"; "Tombstone of Lincoln's Second Son."

9. Lincoln to John D. Johnston, February 23, 1850, *Collected Works*, 2:76–77; Shutes, "Mortality of the Five Lincoln Boys," 3–4; Turner and Turner, *Mary Todd Lincoln*, xvi, 40. Durham also mentioned cholera as well as Marfan syndrome. Durham, "Lincoln's Sons," 70.

10. Temple, "Lincoln in the Census," 137–38; US Census, Mortality Schedule, 1850, Illinois; Baker, *Mary Todd Lincoln*, 136, 138, 143; Epstein, *Lincolns*, 159; Fleischner, *Mrs. Lincoln and Mrs. Keckly*, 169.

11. Lincoln to John D. Johnston, February 23, 1850, *Collected Works*, 2:76–77; Emerson, "'Of Such Is the Kingdom of Heaven'"; Fleischner, *Mrs. Lincoln and Mrs. Keckly*, 169–71; Baker, *Mary Todd Lincoln*, 125–27.

12. Lincoln to John D. Johnston, January 12, 1851, *Collected Works*, 2:97; David Davis to Sarah Davis, May 17, 1852, David Davis Papers, box 8, folder B-9, ALPL.

13. "The Parent and the Politician"; Lincoln to Anson G. Henry, July 4, 1860, *Collected Works*, 4:82; Randall, *Lincoln's Sons*, 58; Durham, "Lincoln's Sons," 70.

14. Mary to Rhoda White, May 2, 1868, Turner and Turner, *Mary Todd Lincoln*, 475; Shutes, "Mortality of the Five Lincoln Boys," 6; Clinton, *Mrs. Lincoln*, 88–89; Epstein, *Lincolns*, 165–66; Baker, *Mary Todd Lincoln*, 270.

15. Hutchinson, "What Was Tad Lincoln's Speech Problem?," 35–51 (summarized 49–51).

16. Mary to Ozias M. Hatch, February 28, 1859, Turner and Turner, *Mary Todd Lincoln*, 53; Randall, *Lincoln's Sons*, 44–45; Goff, *Robert Todd Lincoln*, 10.

17. Lincoln to John D. Johnston, August 31, 1851, *Collected Works*, 2:110; *Illinois Journal*, January 14, 1854, Lincoln Log, January 12, 1854; William H. Herndon to Lyman Trumbull, March 2, 1857, cited in the Lincoln Log, March 2, 1857; Lincoln to Mary, March 4, 1860, *Collected Works Supplement*, 49.

18. Shutes, *Lincoln and the Doctors*, 54; Bailhache, "Abraham Lincoln as I Remember Him"; Temple, *Dr. Anson G. Henry*, 7–9; Temple, "A. W. French"; Lincoln to John T. Stuart, January 20, 1841, *Collected Works*, 1:228.

19. Pratt, *Personal Finances*, 151–53; McAndrew, *Stories of Springfield*, 53–56. The information was previously published in the *State Journal-Register* (Springfield, IL), May 7, 2006, and the *Chicago Times Magazine*, February 11, 2007.

20. Hirschhorn, Feldman, and Greaves, "Abraham Lincoln's Blue Pills," 319–22; Schroeder-Lein, *Encyclopedia of Civil War Medicine*, 58; Ward Hill Lamon interview, Wilson and Davis, *Herndon's Informants*, 466; Henry C. Whitney to Herndon, August 27, 1887, Wilson and Davis, *Herndon's Informants*, 631.

21. Hirschhorn, Feldman, and Greaves, "Abraham Lincoln's Blue Pills," 315–19, 323–26.

22. Schroeder-Lein, *Encyclopedia of Civil War Medicine*, 211–12; Hirschhorn, Feldman, and Greaves, "Abraham Lincoln's Blue Pills," 328; Marcotty, "Mercury in Lincoln's Medicine."

23. Ward Hill Lamon interview, Wilson and Davis, *Herndon's Informants*, 466; Frances Todd Wallace interview, ibid., 485.

24. Shutes, *Lincoln and the Doctors*, 65; Sotos, *Physical Lincoln*, 88; Henry C. Whitney to Herndon, August 27, 1887, Wilson and Davis, *Herndon's Informants*, 631; Boritt and Borit, "Lincoln and the Marfan Syndrome," 219.

25. Brooks, *Washington, D.C.*, 199–200; Shutes, *Lincoln and the Doctors*, 67–68; Sotos, *Physical Lincoln*, 89–90; Boritt and Borit, "Lincoln and the Marfan Syndrome," 220.

3. The Lincoln Family in Washington, DC, 1861–65

1. White, *Eloquent President*, 3–22; Searcher, *Lincoln's Journey to Greatness*, entire book but especially 60, 95–96, 113, 122; Burlingame, *Abraham Lincoln*, 2:10–12, 16–17, 19, 22–24, 26–29, 36.

2. Newspaper reporter, December 14, 1860, McClintock, *Lincoln and the Decision for War*, 87–88; Joshua Speed interview, Wilson and Davis, *Herndon's Informants*, 475.

3. McClintock, *Lincoln and the Decision for War*, 187–253; Fessenden to Home, March 17, 1861, Fessenden, *Life and Public Services*, 1:127; Burlingame,

Abraham Lincoln, 2:108, 115; McPherson, *Tried by War*, 14; Crofts, *Secession Crisis Enigma*, 138; Donald, *"We Are Lincoln Men,"* 103.

4. Grimsley, "Six Months," 55; Orville H. Browning to Lincoln, March 26, 1861, Donald, *"We Are Lincoln Men,"* 114; John G. Nicolay to Therena Bates, March 31 and April 2, 1861, Burlingame, *With Lincoln in the White House*, 32.

5. Nicolay to Bates, March 20, 1861, Burlingame, *With Lincoln in the White House*, 31; Grimsley, "Six Months," 54–55; Furgurson, *Freedom Rising*, 29–30, 35–36, 59; Mary to Hannah Shearer, March 28, 1861, Turner and Turner, *Mary Todd Lincoln*, 81; Elmer Ellsworth to Charles H. Spafford, [March 1861], Ephraim Elmer Ellsworth Papers, SC 455, folder 3, ALPL.

6. Grimsley, "Six Months," 51.

7. Lincoln endorsement, February 15, 1863, L. Richards to Edwin M. Stanton, National Archives, Record Group 92, Records of the Office of the Quartermaster General, 1792–1929, box 886 (old); *History of the Medical Society*, 248; US Census, 1860, Washington, DC.

8. Goff, *Robert Todd Lincoln*, 47.

9. Frances Seward Diary, August 31, 1861, Lincoln Log.

10. Miers, *Lincoln Day by Day*, 3:60, 63–64; Randall, *Lincoln's Sons*, 91; Mary to Elizabeth Todd Grimsley, September 29, 1861, Turner and Turner, *Mary Todd Lincoln*, 104–6; Mary to Hannah Shearer, October 6, 1861, Turner and Turner, *Mary Todd Lincoln*, 108; Schroeder-Lein, *Encyclopedia of Civil War Medicine*, 192–93, 221–23.

11. Samuel P. Heintzelmann Journal, January 26, 1862, Lincoln Log; Keckley, *Behind the Scenes*, 98, 100–102; John Nicolay to Therena Bates, February 11, 1862, Burlingame, *With Lincoln in the White House*, 69; Lincoln Log, February 7–8, 10–15, 19–20. Keckley's name has generally been spelled with a second *e*, as it appears on her book. Jennifer Fleischner discovered that Keckly spelled it herself without the second *e*. It will be spelled Keckly's way in the text. Fleischner, *Mrs. Lincoln and Mrs. Keckly*, 7.

12. Randall, *Lincoln's Sons*, 99; Sotos, *Physical Lincoln*, 143. Other citations will be given as the malady is discussed. For more on MEN2B, see chapter 4.

13. Burlingame, *Abraham Lincoln*, 2: 298.

14. Durham, "Lincoln's Sons," 70. For more on Marfan syndrome, see chapter 4.

15. Shutes, "Mortality of the Five Lincoln Boys," 6; Durham, "Lincoln's Sons," 70; Baker, *Mary Todd Lincoln*, 209.

16. Schroeder-Lein, *Encyclopedia of Civil War Medicine*, 310; Shutes, "Mortality of the Five Lincoln Boys," 5.

17. Bilious fever: Epstein, *Lincolns*, 362; Durham, "Lincoln's Sons," 70. Malaria: Durham, "Lincoln's Sons," 70; Turner and Turner, *Mary Todd Lincoln*, xvi, 121; Evans, *Mrs. Abraham Lincoln*, 140.

18. Schroeder-Lein, *Encyclopedia of Civil War Medicine*, 192–93; Evans, *Mrs. Abraham Lincoln*, 140; Shutes, "Mortality of the Five Lincoln Boys," 5–6.

19. Shutes, "Mortality of the Five Lincoln Boys," 5–6; Shutes, *Lincoln and the Doctors*, 81; Epstein, *Lincolns*, 366; Pearson, "Tragic Deaths," 234.

20. Three newspapers in Shutes, "Mortality of the Five Lincoln Boys," 5; Baker, *Mary Todd Lincoln*, 209; Fleischner, *Mrs. Lincoln and Mrs. Keckly*, 230; Goodwin, *Team of Rivals*, 418–21.

21. Schroeder-Lein, *Encyclopedia of Civil War Medicine*, 309–11; Mayo Clinic, "Typhoid Fever"; Rafuse, "Typhoid and Tumult"; Baker, *Mary Todd Lincoln*, 208–9; Epstein, *Lincolns*, 370; Boyden, *Echoes from Hospital*, 54; Burlingame, *Abraham Lincoln*, 2:298.

22. Keckley, *Behind the Scenes*, 103, 106–8; Nicolay journal, February 20, 1862, Burlingame, *With Lincoln in the White House*, 71; Burlingame, *Abraham Lincoln*, 2:298–300.

23. Keckley, *Behind the Scenes*, 104–5; Elizabeth P. Edwards to Julia Edwards Baker, March 1 and 2, 1862, Elizabeth Parker Todd Edwards Papers, SC 445, ALPL; Randall, *Lincoln's Sons*, 101; Turner and Turner, *Mary Todd Lincoln*, 122; Baker, *Mary Todd Lincoln*, 212; Browning, *Diary*, 1:530–31; Burlingame, *Oral History*, 130–31; Bates, *Diary*, 236; Nicolay journal, February 20, 1862, Burlingame, *With Lincoln in the White House*, 71; Lincoln to Dorothea Dix, February 19, 1862, Emory University, Atlanta, GA, Lincoln Log; Boyden, *Echoes from Hospital*, 14–18, 24, 52–54, 70–71.

24. Boyden, *Echoes from Hospital*, 54–60, 77–79; Holst, "'One of the Best Women,'" 15–16; Browning, *Diary*, 1:608; Helm, *True Story of Mary*, 226–27.

25. *Washington Star*, March 20, 1862, Lincoln Log; Lincoln to Mrs. Irvin McDowell, March 21, 1862, *Collected Works*, 5:168; Keckley, *Behind the Scenes*, 116, 181; French, *Witness*, 392; Bayne, *Tad Lincoln's Father*, 204–5; Mary to Mrs. Charles Eames, July 26, 1862, Turner and Turner, *Mary Todd Lincoln*, 130.

26. Elizabeth P. Edwards to Julia Edwards Baker, March 1 and 2, 1862, Edwards Papers, SC 445, ALPL; Lincoln to Tad, March 10, 1862, *Collected Works*, 5:154.

27. Browning, *Diary*, 1:540, 542–43.

28. Strong, *Diary*, 218; Mary Todd Lincoln interview, Wilson and Davis, *Herndon's Informants*, 360; John Hay to Herndon, September 5, 1866, Wilson and Davis, *Herndon's Informants*, 331; Carpenter, *Inner Life*,

32–34, 317; Brooks, *Washington, D.C.*, 246; Stoddard, *Inside the White House*, 149.

29. Chase to Nettie, May 7, 1862, Salmon P. Chase, *Papers*, 1:336; Symonds, *Lincoln and His Admirals*, 147, 321.

30. Lincoln Log, July 5, 1862; Browning, *Diary*, 1:559.

31. Chase, *Papers*, 1:375; Lincoln Log, September 13 and 25, 1862; "Testimonial for Isachar Zacharie," *Collected Works*, 5:436.

32. John H. Littlefield to Herndon, December 11, 1866, Wilson and Davis, *Herndon's Informants*, 514–15; Shutes, *Lincoln and the Doctors*, 88–89.

33. Brooks, "Personal Reminiscences," 562–63; Brooks, *Washington, D.C.*, 3, 9, 15; French, *Witness*, 416–17.

34. French, *Witness*, 418; Lincoln Log, March 29, 1863; Symonds, *Lincoln and His Admirals*, 209.

35. Brooks, "Personal Reminiscences," 673; Turner and Turner, *Mary Todd Lincoln*, 152; Lincoln to Mary, June 11 and 15, 1863, *Collected Works*, 6:260, 277; French, *Witness*, 422.

36. Boyden, *Echoes from Hospital*, 142–44; Clark, "Abraham Lincoln in the National Capital," 72; *New York Times*, July 3, 1863; Lincoln to Robert, July 3, 1863, *Collected Works*, 6:314; Clinton, *Mrs. Lincoln*, 202–4, 221; Fleischner, *Mrs. Lincoln and Mrs. Keckly*, 260–62; Helm, *True Story of Mary*, 250.

37. Lincoln to Robert C. Schenck, July 23, 1863, *Collected Works*, 6:345–46; Lincoln to Mary, July 28, August 8, September 3, 20, 21, 22, 1863, ibid., 353, 371, 431, 469, 471, 474; Mary to Lincoln, September 22, 1863, Turner and Turner, *Mary Todd Lincoln*, 158; Lincoln Log, September 28, 1863.

38. Lincoln Log, November 18, 1863; Turner and Turner, *Mary Todd Lincoln*, 158; Lincoln to Edward Everett, November 20, 1863, *Collected Works*, 7:24; Randall, *Lincoln's Sons*, 128–29; Shutes, *Lincoln and the Doctors*, 87; Goldman and Schmalstieg, "Abraham Lincoln's Gettysburg Illness," 108; Centers for Disease Control, "Smallpox Disease Overview"; *Washington Chronicle*, November 28, 1863, Lincoln Log.

39. Goldman and Schmalstieg, "Abraham Lincoln's Gettysburg Illness," 108; Basler, "Did President Lincoln Give the Smallpox," 281; Shutes, *Lincoln and the Doctors*, 85; Dennett, *Lincoln and the Civil War*, 122–28; Lincoln to William H. Seward, November 27, 1863, *Collected Works Supplement*, 211; Lincoln Log, November 25–27, 1863.

40. Lincoln Log, November 30, December 1, 3–4, 10–12, 14–15, 1863; French, *Witness*, 439; Mary to Lincoln, December 4, 1863, Turner and Turner, *Mary Todd Lincoln*, 159; Lincoln to Mary, December 4, 5, 6, 7, 1863, *Collected Works*, 7:34–35; Welles, *Diary*, 1:485.

41. Lincoln Log, November 21, 1863; Fessenden, *Life and Public Services*, 1:267; Strong, *Diary*, 383; Holzer, *Lincoln's White House Secretary*, 305;

Browning, *Diary*, 1:650–51; Basler, "Did President Lincoln Give the Smallpox"; Lincoln to Robert, January 19, 1864, *Collected Works*, 7:137; Goldman and Schmalstieg, "Abraham Lincoln's Gettysburg Illness," 108–10.

42. *Sacramento Daily Union*, February 4, 1864; Bernard, "Lincoln and the Music of the Civil War," 169; Lincoln to Mary, January 7, 1864, *Collected Works*, 7:112; French, *Witness*, 443; Lincoln Log, January 26 and February 9, 1864.

43. Lincoln to Salmon P. Chase, February 13 and 15, 1864, *Collected Works*, 7:182, 184; Mary to Daniel E. Sickles, February 20, 1864, Turner and Turner, *Mary Todd Lincoln*, 169; French, *Witness*, 447–49.

44. Lincoln to Benjamin F. Butler, April 11, 1864, *Collected Works*, 7:293; *Washington Star*, April 16, 1864, Lincoln Log; Lincoln to Mary, April 28, 1864, *Collected Works*, 7:320; Lincoln to Robert K. Stone, May 26, 1864, T. Schwartz, "Whither *The Collected Works*," 55; Mary to Mary Jane Welles, May 27, 1864, Turner and Turner, *Mary Todd Lincoln*, 176.

45. Lincoln Log, June 21 and 23, 1864; Welles, *Diary*, 2:61; French, *Witness*, 456; Mary to George D. Ramsay, July 20, 1864, and to Abram Wakeman, September 23, 1864, Turner and Turner, *Mary Todd Lincoln*, 177, 180; Lincoln to Robert, October 11, 1864, *Collected Works*, 8:44.

46. French, *Witness*, 463; Shutes, *Lincoln and the Doctors*, 108–9; Browning, *Diary*, 2:7–8; Joshua Speed interview, Wilson and Davis, *Herndon's Informants*, 157.

47. Swisshelm letter from Washington, July 11, 1865, reprinted in *St. Cloud (Minnesota) Democrat*, August 3, 1865, reprinted in Larsen, *Crusader and Feminist*, 300.

48. Welles, *Diary*, 2:257; Lincoln Log, March 13–16, 1865.

49. Mary to Charles Sumner, March 23, 1865, Turner and Turner, *Mary Todd Lincoln*, 209; Welles, *Diary*, 2:264.

50. Barnes, "With Lincoln," 521–22; Maj. William L. James to Lincoln, March 24, 1865, with Lincoln endorsement, March 24, 1865, *Collected Works*, 8:373; Charles R. Penrose to Edwin M. Stanton, March 24, 1865, *Collected Works*, 8:373.

51. Lincoln Log, March 26–April 8, 1865; Porter, *Campaigning with Grant*, 412–14; Baker, *Mary Todd Lincoln*, 238–40; Barnes, "With Lincoln," 524, 743; Lincoln to Mary, April 2, 1865, *Collected Works*, 8:384; Mary to Abram Wakeman, April 4, 1865, Turner and Turner, *Mary Todd Lincoln*, 213.

52. Barnes, "With Lincoln," 745, 748–49.

53. Chambrun, "Personal Recollections," 29–31; Carpenter, *Inner Life*, 287–89; Cornelia Hancock to Sister, April 11, 1865, Jacquette, *Letters*, 170; Burlingame, *Abraham Lincoln*, 2:796–97; Shutes, *Lincoln and the*

Doctors, 99–101; Boritt and Borit, "Lincoln and the Marfan Syndrome," 223–24; Keckley, *Behind the Scenes*, 171–73.

54. Welles, *Diary*, 2:278; Mary to Charles Sumner, April 11, 1865, Turner and Turner, *Mary Todd Lincoln*, 217; Mary to Ulysses S. Grant, April 13, 1865, Turner and Turner, *Mary Todd Lincoln*, 219.

4. Lincoln and the Medical Bandwagon

1. For some of the rarely mentioned diagnoses, see Pearson, "Abraham Lincoln—Health"; and Miller, "Pay Attention."

2. Borrit and Borit, "Lincoln and the Marfan Syndrome," 212; Lattimer, "Danger in Claiming," 40, 46; Micozzi, "When the Patient Is Abraham Lincoln," 35.

3. For more information on Marfan syndrome, see the MedicineNet website at www.medicinenet.com/marfan_syndrome/page2.htm (accessed 01/12/2011). There are other sites, but this one was straightforward. Reilly, *Abraham Lincoln's DNA*, 4.

4. Gordon, "Abraham Lincoln—A Medical Appraisal," 252–53; Boritt and Borit, "Lincoln and the Marfan Syndrome," 212–13; Lattimer, "Danger in Claiming," 43.

5. H. Schwartz, "Abraham Lincoln and the Marfan Syndrome"; Boritt and Borit, "Lincoln and the Marfan Syndrome," 213; Lattimer, "Danger in Claiming," 40, 43, 46.

6. Temple, "Lincoln in the Census," 138; Durham, "Lincoln's Sons," 67–68; Boritt and Borit, "Lincoln and the Marfan Syndrome," 214, 216–17; "Why Abe Was No Beauty"; "Doctor Claims Lincoln Had Fatal Malady."

7. Lattimer, "Lincoln Did Not Have the Marfan Syndrome," 1805–7; Boritt and Borit, "Lincoln and the Marfan Syndrome," 218; Reilly, *Abraham Lincoln's DNA*, 11.

8. H. Schwartz, "Abraham Lincoln and Cardiac Decompensation"; Boritt and Borit, "Lincoln and the Marfan Syndrome," 214, 219–22; Lattimer, "Lincoln Did Not Have the Marfan Syndrome," 1809–12.

9. Lattimer, "Lincoln Did Not Have the Marfan Syndrome"; Lattimer, "Danger in Claiming."

10. Brown, "Is Lincoln Earliest Recorded Case"; Sotos, *Physical Lincoln*, 26, 27, 119–20.

11. Brown, "Is Lincoln Earliest Recorded Case"; Sotos, *Physical Lincoln*, 15, 125–26.

12. Sotos, *Physical Lincoln*, chapter 14 (bumpy lips); 15, 138–39 (constipation); 187–93 (muscle tone); 194–202 (asymmetrical head); 197.

13. Ibid., 149–51, 158, 175–79, 221; Brown, "Is Lincoln Earliest Recorded Case."

14. Sotos, *Physical Lincoln*, 175–79.

15. Brown, "Is Lincoln Earliest Recorded Case."
16. Sotos, *Physical Lincoln*, 221.
17. "Study Traces Gene Defect in Abe's Family"; "Research Hints at an Ailment in Lincoln"; Prokopowicz, *Did Lincoln Own Slaves?*, 194; "Mutant Gene Shatters Nerves."
18. Kaye, *Double Helix*, 38–40; Robinson, *Genetics for Dummies*, 83–95. *Genetics for Dummies* provides a useful overview for nonspecialists.
19. Robinson, *Genetics for Dummies*, 86, 93–94, 269; Davidson, "Abraham Lincoln and the DNA Controversy," 13, 15.
20. Brown, "Is Lincoln Earliest Recorded Case"; Reilly, *Abraham Lincoln's DNA*, 5–6; Colimore, "Lincoln's 'Shroud of Turin'"; Craughwell, *Stealing Lincoln's Body*, 194–97.
21. Micozzi, "When the Patient Is Abraham Lincoln," 36, 40; Davidson, "Abraham Lincoln and the DNA Controversy," 3–4.
22. Micozzi, "When the Patient Is Abraham Lincoln," 36–40; Davidson, "Abraham Lincoln and the DNA Controversy," 6–8, 21, 24; McKusick, "Advisory Statement," 44–46.
23. Micozzi, "When the Patient Is Abraham Lincoln," 36; Davidson, "Abraham Lincoln and the DNA Controversy," 6, 10, 15–16, 18; Reilly, *Abraham Lincoln's DNA*, 9.
24. Brown, "Is Lincoln Earliest Recorded Case"; Colimore, "Lincoln's 'Shroud of Turin'"; Todt, "Test of Lincoln's DNA Sought"; Bixler, "DNA Test."
25. Biscuit Factory, *Lincoln's Secret Killer?*
26. Lincoln Biohistory Study Group, agendas and notes, provided by T. Schwartz, member of Ethics Panel.
27. Monroe, "Review," 140; Donald, *"We Are Lincoln Men,"* 35–36; Smith, "Lincoln Scholarship," 65; Prokopowicz, *Did Lincoln Own Slaves?*, 48.
28. Tripp, *Intimate World*, xxxii; Smith, "Lincoln Scholarship," 61.
29. Tripp, *Intimate World*, xxvii–xxix.
30. Ibid., xxx; Robbins, "Writer Asserts"; Prokopowicz, *Did Lincoln Own Slaves?*, 47; Steers, *Lincoln Legends*, 125–26.
31. Baker, "Introduction," xiv, xvi; Steers, *Lincoln Legends*, 126.
32. David Turnham interview, Wilson and Davis, *Herndon's Informants*, 120–21; Tripp, *Intimate World*, 31–32, 34–36; Steers, *Lincoln Legends*, 128–31; Blum, review of Tripp.
33. Tripp, *Intimate World*, 20, 126–27; Prokopowicz, *Did Lincoln Own Slaves?*, 49; Turner, "Editor's Introduction," 156; Steers, *Lincoln Legends*, 127; Monroe, "Review," 140.
34. Speed, "Incidents in the Early Life of A. Lincoln," SC 1443-A, ALPL, also published in Wilson and Davis, *Herndon's Informants*, 589–90; Tripp, *Intimate World*, 126–27; Burlingame, *Abraham Lincoln*, 1:131; White, *A. Lincoln*, 79–80.

35. Tripp, *Intimate World*, 126–27, 133.
36. Ibid., chapter 1; Donald, *"We Are Lincoln Men,"* 140–46; Epstein, *Lincolns*, 377; Johnson, "Did Abraham Lincoln Sleep with His Body-guard?," entire article but especially 43, 51–53.
37. Tripp, *Intimate World*, 47, 53, 62; Wilson and Davis, *Herndon's Informants*, 17–18; Steers, *Lincoln Legends*, 133.
38. Hanchett, "Abraham Lincoln and the Tripp Thesis," part 4, 10–11; Smith, "Lincoln Scholarship," 62; Shenk, *Lincoln's Melancholy*, 34.
39. Donald, *"We Are Lincoln Men,"* 35–36; Prokopowicz, *Did Lincoln Own Slaves?*, 50; Burlingame, *Abraham Lincoln*, 1:326–27; Whitney, *Life on the Circuit*, 559.
40. Goodwin, *Team of Rivals*, 33; Shenk, *Lincoln's Melancholy*, 33; Donald, *"We Are Lincoln Men,"* 35–36; Tripp, *Intimate World*, xxix, 62, 128; Prokopowicz, *Did Lincoln Own Slaves?*, 50.
41. James M. Taylor to Isabella Low, September 6 and October 19, 1862, both folder 2; James M. Taylor and John Y. Taylor to Mary Bater, December 4, 1862, folder 2; James M. Taylor to Isabella Low, March 7, 1863, folder 3; James M. Taylor diary, April 29, 1863, folder 1; James M. Taylor to James and Mary Bater, May 1, 1863, and to Isabella Low, May 3, 1863, both folder 3; James M. Taylor to probably Isabella Low, February 6, 1864, folder 4, all in box 1, Taylor Family (James M.) Papers, ALPL. This collection is a good example of common practices.
42. Burlingame, *Abraham Lincoln*, 1:327; Sarah Bush Johnston Lincoln interview, Wilson and Davis, *Herndon's Informants*, 108; John Hay to Herndon, September 5, 1866, Wilson and Davis, *Herndon's Informants*, 331.
43. Baker, "Introduction," xiv, xxi–xxii; Chesson, "Enthusiastic Endorsement," 238–46.
44. Hanchett, "Abraham Lincoln and the Tripp Thesis," part 4, 11–13.
45. Burlingame, "Respectful Dissent," 225–38.
46. Blum, review of Tripp; Steers, *Lincoln Legends*, 128–31; Pinsker, "Review"; Smith, "Lincoln Scholarship," 62.
47. Monroe, "Review," 141; Smith, "Lincoln Scholarship," 61; Steers, *Lincoln Legends*, 127, 149; Hathaway, "Review"; Prokopowicz, *Did Lincoln Own Slaves?*, 51; Tripp, *Intimate World*, xxix (Burlingame quote).
48. Blum, review of Tripp; Pinsker, "Review," 1442; Steers, *Lincoln Legends*, 128; Johnson, "Did Abraham Lincoln Sleep with His Bodyguard?," 42.

5. Lincoln and Medical Matters during the Civil War

1. Spiegal, *A. Lincoln*.
2. Adams, *Doctors in Blue*, 4–5; Schroeder-Lein, *Encyclopedia of Civil War Medicine*, 108, 181–82.

3. Schroeder-Lein, *Encyclopedia of Civil War Medicine*, 313–18, 333–35. Each article has a bibliography.

4. Ibid., 315; Lincoln, *Collected Works Supplement*, 76–77; Maxwell, *Lincoln's Fifth Wheel*, 8, 12–13, 19; Strong, *Diary*, 159.

5. John G. Nicolay to Alexander D. Bache, July 31, 1861, Burlingame, *With Lincoln in the White House*, 53; Lincoln to John C. Frémont, August 2, 1861, *Collected Works*, 4:469; Lincoln to Winfield Scott, September 30, 1861, *Collected Works*, 4:543; Maxwell, *Lincoln's Fifth Wheel*, 103–4; Schroeder-Lein, *Encyclopedia of Civil War Medicine*, 333.

6. Strong, *Diary*, 186–88, 204.

7. Brooks, *Washington, D.C.*, 37; Lincoln to Benjamin B. French, July 1, 1863, *Collected Works*, 6:312–13; Lincoln to Edward Bates, November 13, 1863, *Collected Works*, 7:12.

8. Adams, *Doctors in Blue*, 30–32; Schroeder-Lein, *Encyclopedia of Civil War Medicine*, 123–24; Hammond, *Statement of the Causes*. Blustein, *Preserve Your Love for Science* is a good biography of Hammond.

9. Strong, *Diary*, 385, 389, 394, 396; Lincoln to Mrs. William A. Hammond, August 2, 1864, *Collected Works*, 7:474–75; Lincoln endorsement, August 18, 1864, *Collected Works*, 7:503; Schroeder-Lein, *Encyclopedia of Civil War Medicine*, 36.

10. These are just a small sample of the requests Lincoln received and acted upon. From *Collected Works*: Lincoln to Lorenzo Thomas, August 29, 1861, 4:503; Lincoln to Zachariah Chandler, September 7, 1861, 4:512; Lincoln to Simon Cameron, November 7, December 12 and 13, 1861, 5:17, 65, 67; Lincoln to Edwin M. Stanton, March 1 and 25, 1862, 5:140, 171. Worthington, "Open Polar Sea."

11. Lincoln to Archbishop John J. Hughes, October 21, 1861, *Collected Works*, 4:559; Lincoln to Rev. F. M. Magrath, October 30, 1861, ibid., 5:8–9; First Annual Message, December 3, 1861, ibid., 5:40.

12. J. Christian Miller to Lincoln, June 3, 1862; C. L. (or S.) Macreading to Lincoln, June 13, 1862; Benjamin N. Reed to Lincoln, May 16, 1862, all in Letters to Abraham Lincoln, SC 914-E, ALPL. There are also other letters about the hospital chaplaincy in this collection. Browning, *Diary*, 1:591; Phineas D. Gurley to Lincoln, December 6, 1862, Phineas D. Gurley Letters, SC 616, ALPL; Lincoln to William A. Hammond, May 1, 1863, *Collected Works*, 6:194.

13. Lincoln memorandum, January 6, 1863, *Collected Works*, 6:41; Lincoln to Stanton, January 21, 1863, *Collected Works Supplement*, 175, and September 5, 1864, *Collected Works*, 7:537–38.

14. Lincoln to Stanton, May 22 and August 2, 1862, *Collected Works*, 5:229–30, 367; Lincoln to Hammond, August 19, 1862, ibid., 5:382–83; Lincoln to Lorenzo Thomas, ca. August 29, 1862, ibid., 5:400; Lincoln

to Stanton, July 27 and October 30, 1863, ibid., 6:351–52, and *Collected Works Supplement*, 208; George, "Lincoln to Stanton"; Lincoln to Benjamin F. Butler, September 27, 1864, *Collected Works*, 8:25.

15. Lowry and Welsh, *Tarnished Scalpels*, 54–58, 110–17, 149–59, 215–20; Lowry, *Merciful Lincoln*, 40–41, 44–45; Lincoln to Andrew G. Curtin, August 18, 1862 (and associated documents), *Collected Works*, 5:380; Lincoln to Joseph Holt, June 18, 1863 and May 5, 1864, *Collected Works*, 6:285–86, 7:332; Lincoln to Stanton, January 12, 1863, *Collected Works*, 6:55.

16. Spiegal, *A. Lincoln*, chapter 13; Lincoln to John P. Gray, September 10 and 13, 1863, *Collected Works*, 6:437–38, 443; Statement, October 7, 1863, *Collected Works*, 6:505; Lincoln to John G. Foster, August 28, October 15 and 17, 1863, *Collected Works*, 6:419, 514, 522.

17. Lincoln to Stanton, March 18, 1864, *Collected Works*, 7:255.

18. Lincoln to Hammond, May 22, 1862, ibid., 5:228–29; Salmon P. Chase to Lincoln, September 28, 1862, and endorsements, ibid., 444–45; Lincoln Log, September 21, 1862; Strong, *Diary*, 304; Lincoln testimonials, September 22 and 23, 1862, *Collected Works*, 5:436, and *Collected Works Supplement*, 152–53; Lincoln to Senate and House of Representatives, April 23, 1864, *Collected Works*, 7:311.

19. Lincoln to Medical Director, March 30, 1862, *Collected Works Supplement*, 127–28; Lincoln to Hammond, June 4, 1862, *Collected Works*, 5:259; Lincoln endorsements, October 17, 1863, and October 20, 1864, *Collected Works Supplement*, 206, and *Collected Works*, 8:54–55; Lincoln to Stanton, October 15, 1863, *Collected Works*, 6:516; Harvey, "Wisconsin Woman's Picture," 240–55.

20. Moses P. Rice et al. to Lincoln, ca. March 3, 1863, Lincoln Collection, box 11, ALPL.

21. Boyden, *Echoes from Hospital*, 57–60, 77–78, 92, 94–95, 119, 131–32; Lincoln to Dorothea Dix, May 4, 1862, *Collected Works Supplement*, 132; Lincoln to Stanton, *Collected Works*, 5:326–27. The visit with Browning may have been on May 18, 1862. Browning, *Diary*, 1:546.

22. Lincoln Log, July 31 and August 3, 1861, December 25, 1862, and May 24, 1863; *Chicago Times*, October 10, 1862; Brooks, *Washington, D.C.*, 54; Chambrun, "Personal Recollections," 29–31; Holst, "One of the Best Women," 18; Orton, "Eyewitness Account"; Brinton, *Personal Memoirs*, 265.

23. Mary to Mary Jane Welles, May 27, 1864, Turner and Turner, *Mary Todd Lincoln*, 176; Lincoln to Hiram P. Barney, August 16, 1862, *Collected Works*, 5:377–78; *Washington Evening Star*, August 29, 1862; Lincoln Log, October 4, 1862; Clark, "Abraham Lincoln in the National Capital," 39–40; Mary to Thomas W. Sweney, April 1863, Turner and

Turner, *Mary Todd Lincoln*, 149–50; Mary to Mrs. Agen, August 10, 1864, Turner and Turner, *Mary Todd Lincoln*, 179; Boyden, *Echoes from Hospital*, 98–99.

24. Lincoln to Richard Yates, February 3, 1864, *Collected Works*, 7:167; Lincoln Log, June 16, 1862, April 1 and September 8, 1863, March 8 and November 4, 1864; Lincoln to Stanton, September 27, 1863, *Collected Works*, 5:443; Carpenter, *Inner Life*, 107–8, 140; Benjamin B. French to Lincoln, August 19, 1863, *Collected Works*, 6:397–98; Lincoln to Stanton, October 13, 1862, *Collected Works Supplement*, 157.

25. Spiegel, *A. Lincoln*, 273. From *Collected Works*: Lincoln to Joseph Holt (various documents), 7:227; Lincoln to John P. Gray, April 25, 1864, 7:313–14; Lincoln to Edward Bates, June 11, 1862, 5:266; Lincoln endorsements, June 16, 1863, September 5, 7, and 23, 1864, 6:280, 7:538, 541–42, 8:19; Lincoln to Joseph Holt, April 14, 1864, 7:298–99.

26. From *Collected Works*: Lincoln to Hammond, September 18, 1862, 5:429; Lincoln to Stanton, May 29, 1862, September 2 and October 16, 1863, June 1864 (?), 5:249, 6:429, 520, 7:372–73; Lincoln to Hannah Armstrong, September 18, 1863, 6:462; Lincoln to Joseph K. Barnes, February 25, 1864, 7:203; Lincoln to Stanton, May 10 and August 9, 1864, 7:335, 524–25.

27. From *Collected Works*: Lincoln to William W. Morris, March 13, 1863, 6:135; Lincoln to Stanton, July 28 and December 19, 1863, February 20, 1864, 6:353, 7:80, 195; Lincoln endorsement, August 30, November 11 and 17, 1864, February 13, 1865, 7:524, 8:103, 112, 296; Lincoln to Charles W. Hill, February 4, 1865, 8:259; Lincoln to Alexander H. Stephens, February 10, 1865, 8:287.

28. From *Collected Works*: Lincoln to Edwin D. Morgan, September 6, 1862, 5:408; Lincoln to Stanton, January 31, September 19 and 23, 1863, 6:86, 490, 477; Lincoln to Stanton, October 21, 1862, August 28, 1863, April 8, 1864, 5:471, 6:419, 7:291; Lincoln to Hiram Barney, May 9, 1864, 7:332–33.

29. Lincoln, "Annual Message," December 6, 1864, ibid., 8:147.

30. Rafuse, "Typhoid and Tumult."

31. Lincoln Log, March 10, 1862, July 5, 1863; Lincoln to Ulysses S. Grant, October 8, 1862, *Collected Works*, 5:453; Lincoln to Stanton, December 16, 1863 and December 21, 1864, *Collected Works*, 7:74, 8:175; Welles, *Diary*, 2:94.

32. Carpenter, *Inner Life*, 17–18; Basler, "Did President Lincoln Give the Smallpox," 282–84; Goodwin, *Team of Rivals*, 720–21, 724–25, 744–45.

33. Schroeder-Lein, *Encyclopedia of Civil War Medicine*, 269–70; Kramer, "Lincoln at the Fair," 349; Lincoln to Ladies, October 26, 1863, *Collected Works*, 6:539; Lincoln to James H. Hoes, December 17, 1863, *Collected Works*, 7:75.

34. Kramer, "Lincoln at the Fair," 347–50, 352–53; telegrams between Lincoln and Alexander Rice, November 8 and 22, 1864, *Collected Works*, 8:96–97; Salmon P. Chase to Lincoln, January 17, 1864, *Collected Works*, 7:187; Lincoln to Edward Everett, February 4, 1864, *Collected Works*, 7:167–68.

35. Lincoln to the New England Kitchen, March 2, 1864, *Collected Works*, 7:220; Lincoln to Mrs. Augustus C. French, May 16, 1864, *Collected Works Supplement*, 242; Lincoln to Mrs. Field, May 31, 1864, *Collected Works*, 7:369; Kramer, "Lincoln at the Fair," 351–52.

36. Lincoln to Ladies . . . Springfield, Massachusetts, December 19, 1864, *Collected Works*, 8:171; Lincoln to Felix Schmedding, May 20, 1864, ibid., 7:354; Lincoln to Alfred Mackay, May 20, 1864, ibid., 7:353.

37. Lincoln's remarks, February 22 and March 18, 1864, ibid., 7:197–98, 253–54; Kramer, "Lincoln at the Fair," 340–42; French, *Witness*, 444–45.

38. Lincoln's address, April 18, 1864, *Collected Works*, 7:301–3; Welles, *Diary*, 2:15.

39. Schroeder-Lein, "Lincoln and the Great Central Sanitary Fair"; Lincoln Log, June 16–17, 1864; "Lincoln's Visit to Philadelphia"; Stillé, *Memorial*, 29–30, 135–36; Lincoln, three speeches, June 16, 1864, *Collected Works*, 7:394–96, 397–98.

40. Lincoln to Benjamin B. French, July 1, 1863, *Collected Works*, 6:312–13.

6. The Assassination of Lincoln

1. Trefousse, "Belated Revelations," 14; Read, "A Hand to Hold," 22; *Who Was Who in America*, s.v. "Leale"; Schroeder-Lein, *Encyclopedia of Civil War Medicine*, 202–3. For general accounts of the assassination, see Hanchett, *Lincoln Murder Conspiracies*; and Steers, *Blood on the Moon*.

2. Trefousse, "Belated Revelations"; Leale, *Lincoln's Last Hours*; Taft, "Notes of the circumstances attending the assassination"; Taft, *Abraham Lincoln's Last Hours*.

3. Trefousse, "Belated Revelations," 15; Leale, *Lincoln's Last Hours*, 4–5, 7, 9–10.

4. Trefousse, "Belated Revelations," 15; Taft, *Abraham Lincoln's Last Hours*.

5. Leale, *Lincoln's Last Hours*, 5–6.

6. Ibid., 6–8; Trefousse, "Belated Revelations," 15; Taft, "Notes of the circumstances attending the assassination," 3–4.

7. Leale, *Lincoln's Last Hours*, 9; Taft, "Notes of the circumstances attending the assassination," 4–5; Taft, *Abraham Lincoln's Last Hours*.

8. Leale, *Lincoln's Last Hours*, 9–10.

9. Ibid., 10; Taft, "Notes of the circumstances attending the assassination," 5.

10. Leale, *Lincoln's Last Hours*, 11–12; Trefousse, "Belated Revelations," 16; Taft, "Notes of the circumstances attending the assassination," 5–6.

11. Leale, *Lincoln's Last Hours*, 13.

12. Taft, "Notes of the circumstances attending the assassination," 7; Kauff-man, *American Brutus*, 449 n. 24; Leale, *Lincoln's Last Hours*, 14.

13. Lattimer, "Wound That Killed Lincoln," 483–86; Taft, "Notes of the circumstances attending the assassination," 8; Welles, *Diary*, 2:287; Kauffman, *American Brutus*, 242; Henry, *Armed Forces Institute of Pathology*, 41–44.

14. Quoted in Lattimer, "Danger in Claiming," 43; Welles, *Diary*, 2:286.

15. Taft, "Notes of the circumstances attending the assassination," 9; Schroeder-Lein, *Encyclopedia of Civil War Medicine*, 99–100; Kunhardt and Kunhardt, *Twenty Days*.

16. Leale, *Lincoln's Last Hours*, 5; Taft, *Abraham Lincoln's Last Hours*; Henry, *Armed Forces Institute of Pathology*, 44.

17. Brown, "Could Modern Medicine," 114.

7. Lincoln's Family after the War

1. Leale, *Lincoln's Last Hours*, 11.

2. Keckley, *Behind the Scenes*, 191–93; Schroeder-Lein and Zuczek, *Andrew Johnson*, 179.

3. Keckley, *Behind the Scenes*, 210. From Turner and Turner, *Mary Todd Lincoln*, see: Mary to Anson G. Henry, July 17, 1865, 259–61, and Mary to Mary Jane Welles, December 29, 1865, 315–16. See also Mary to Eliza Henry, August 31, 1865, 272; Mary to Alexander Williamson, November 11, 1865, 280; Mary to David Davis, December 13, 1865, 304; Mary to Sally Orne, December 24 and 30, 1865, January 4 and 10, 1866, 311, 318, 323; and Mary to Alexander Williamson, January 19 and February 17, 1866, 328, 336, 338.

4. See throughout Turner and Turner, *Mary Todd Lincoln*; Emerson, *Madness*, 35.

5. Mary to Alexander Williamson, August 17 and December 16, 1865, Turner and Turner, *Mary Todd Lincoln*, 264, 308; Mary to Williamson, October 10, 1865, T. Schwartz and Bauer, "Unpublished Mary Todd Lincoln," 10.

6. Robert to David Davis, January 17, 1868, Goff, *Robert Todd Lincoln*, 94.

7. Randall, *Lincoln's Sons*, 198, 200–208.

8. Ibid., 208–10; Mary to Rhoda White, June 8, 1871, Turner and Turner, *Mary Todd Lincoln*, 590; obituary, *Chicago Tribune*, July 16, 1871; obituary, *Illinois State Register*, July 17, 1871.

9. Shutes, "Mortality of the Five Lincoln Boys," 7; Evans, *Mrs. Abraham Lincoln*, 212.

10. Durham, "Lincoln's Sons," 70; Gordon, "Abraham Lincoln," 252; Boritt and Borit, "Lincoln and the Marfan Syndrome," 223; Sotos, *Physical Lincoln*, 115, 143, 145.

11. Turner and Turner, *Mary Todd Lincoln*, 586; Mary to Eliza Slataper, October 4, 1871, ibid., 596; Emerson, *Madness*, 35–36.

12. Emerson, *Madness*, 43–47; Turner and Turner, *Mary Todd Lincoln*, 608–9.

13. Emerson, *Madness*, 54–59, 61, 72–73, 112, 190; Neely and McMurtry, *Insanity File*, 36–37, 133–35; Ross, "Mary Todd Lincoln," 8–11.

14. Baker, *Mary Todd Lincoln*, chapter 11; Emerson, *Madness*, 104–11.

15. Berry, *House of Abraham*, 186; Evans, *Mrs. Abraham Lincoln*, 312.

16. Emerson, *Madness*, 28, 47, 102, 135; O. H. Browning interview in Burlingame, *Oral History*, 3.

17. Baker, *Mary Todd Lincoln*, 334; T. Schwartz, "'My stay on Earth,'" 135; Neely and McMurtry, *Insanity File*, 33; Emerson, *Madness*, 40–42, 206 n. 53; Clinton, *Mrs. Lincoln*, 305.

18. Baker, *Mary Todd Lincoln*, 326; Neely and McMurtry, *Insanity File*, 34–35; Hirschhorn, "Mary Lincoln's 'Suicide Attempt,'" 94–97.

19. Evans, *Mrs. Abraham Lincoln*, 230, 287, 315–18; Baker, *Mary Todd Lincoln*, 331; Neely and McMurtry, *Insanity File*, 32–33, 141; Emerson, *Madness*, 5, 151–53, 187–90.

20. Mary to Myra Bradwell, July 6, 1878, Emerson, *Madness*, 176; Mary to Edward Lewis Baker Jr., October 4, 1879, January 16, June 12, and August 29, 1880, Turner and Turner, *Mary Todd Lincoln*, 690, 694, 699, 701; see also Turner and Turner, *Mary Todd Lincoln*, 618–19, 692–93.

21. Emerson, *Madness*, 131, 192; Mary to Josephine Remann Edwards, October 23, 1881, Turner and Turner, *Mary Todd Lincoln*, 708–9; Hirschhorn and Feldman, "Mary Lincoln's Final Illness," 511, 517–18.

22. Thomas W. Dresser interview, Wilson and Davis, *Herndon's Informants*, 671; Evans, *Mrs. Abraham Lincoln*, 343–44; Turner and Turner, *Mary Todd Lincoln*, 705; Randall, *Lincoln's Sons*, 234–35.

23. Thomas W. Dresser interview, Wilson and Davis, *Herndon's Informants*, 671; Evans, *Mrs. Abraham Lincoln*, 343–44; Emerson, *Madness*, 132; Hirschhorn and Feldman, "Mary Lincoln's Final Illness."

24. Randall, *Lincoln's Sons*, 212, 241, 260; Mary to Eliza Slataper, August(?) 13, 1871, Turner and Turner, *Mary Todd Lincoln*, 592; Emerson, *Madness*, 4, 21, 49.

25. Randall, *Lincoln's Sons*, 257, 259–63; Neely and McMurtry, *Insanity File*, 144.

BIBLIOGRAPHY

Adams, George Worthington. *Doctors in Blue: The Medical History of the Union Army in the Civil War*. New York: Schuman, 1952; reprint, Dayton, OH: Morningside, 1985.

Bach, Jennifer. "Was Mary Todd Lincoln Bipolar?" *Journal of Illinois History* 8 (Winter 2005): 281–94.

Bailhache, Preston H. "Abraham Lincoln as I Remember Him." John E. Boos Papers. SC 2609, Manuscripts Department. Abraham Lincoln Presidential Library, Springfield, IL.

Baker, Jean H. "Introduction." In *The Intimate World of Abraham Lincoln*, by C. A. Tripp. New York: Free Press, 2005. ix–xxiii.

———. *Mary Todd Lincoln: A Biography*. New York: W. W. Norton, 1987.

Barnes, John S. "With Lincoln from Washington to Richmond in 1865." *Appleton's Magazine*, May 1907, 516–24; June 1907, 742–51.

Basler, Roy P. "Did President Lincoln Give the Smallpox to William H. Johnson?" *Huntington Library Quarterly* 35 (May 1972): 279–84.

Bates, Edward. *The Diary of Edward Bates, 1859–1866*. Edited by Howard K. Beale. Washington, DC: US Government Printing Office, 1933.

Bayne, Julia Taft. *Tad Lincoln's Father*. Boston: Little, Brown, 1931; reprint, Lincoln: University of Nebraska Press, 2001.

Bernard, Kenneth A. "Lincoln and the Music of the Civil War (Part XV): Washington Is Gay." *Lincoln Herald* 65 (Winter 1963): 167–77.

Berry, Stephen. *House of Abraham: Lincoln and the Todds, a Family Divided by War*. Boston: Houghton Mifflin, 2007.

Biscuit Factory. *Lincoln's Secret Killer?* National Geographic Television, aired February 2011. DVD.

Bixler, Jennifer Pifer. "DNA Test Could Shed Light on Lincoln's Last Days, Doctor Says." CNN.com. Accessed August 21, 2010. www.cnn.com/2009/health/05/05/lincoln.cancer.pillow.index.html.

Blum, Edward. Review of *The Intimate World of Abraham Lincoln*, by C. A. Tripp. H-Civ War, H-Net Reviews. August 2005. http://www.h-net.org/reviews/showrev.php?id=10810.

Blustein, Bonnie Ellen. *Preserve Your Love for Science: Life of William A. Hammond, American Neurologist*. Cambridge: Cambridge University Press, 1991.

Boritt, Gabor S., and Adam Borit. "Lincoln and the Marfan Syndrome: The Medical Diagnosis of a Historical Figure." *Civil War History* 29 (September 1983): 212–29.

Boyden, Anna L. *Echoes from Hospital and White House: A Record of Mrs. Rebecca R. Pomroy's Experience in War-Times*. Boston: D. Lothrop, 1884.

Brinton, John H. *Personal Memoirs of John H. Brinton, Civil War Surgeon, 1861–1865.* New York: Neale, 1914; reprint, Carbondale: Southern Illinois University Press, 1996.

Brooks, Noah. "Personal Reminiscences of Lincoln." *Scribner's Monthly* 15 (February 1878): 561–69; (March 1878): 673–81.

———. *Washington, D.C., in Lincoln's Time.* Edited by Herbert Mitgang. 1895; reprint, Athens: University of Georgia Press, 1989.

Brown, David. "Could Modern Medicine Have Saved Lincoln?" *Washington Post*, May 21, 2007; reprinted in *Journal of Civil War Medicine* 11 (October–December 2007): 114–15.

———. "Is Lincoln Earliest Recorded Case of Rare Disease?" *Washington Post*, November 26, 2007. www.washingtonpost.com/wp-dyn/content/article/2007/11/25/AR2007112501224_pf.html.

Browning, Orville Hickman. *The Diary of Orville Hickman Browning.* Edited by Theodore Calvin Pease and James G. Randall. 2 vols. Springfield: Illinois State Historical Library, 1925, 1933.

Burlingame, Michael. *Abraham Lincoln: A Life.* 2 vols. Baltimore, Md.: Johns Hopkins University Press, 2008.

———. *An Oral History of Abraham Lincoln: John G. Nicolay's Interviews and Essays.* Carbondale: Southern Illinois University Press, 1996.

———. "A Respectful Dissent." In *The Intimate World of Abraham Lincoln*, by C. A. Tripp. New York: Free Press, 2005. 225–38.

———, ed. *With Lincoln in the White House: Letters, Memoranda, and Other Writings of John G. Nicolay, 1860–1865.* Carbondale: Southern Illinois University Press, 2000.

Carpenter, Frank B. *The Inner Life of Abraham Lincoln: Six Months at the White House.* New York: Hurd and Houghton, 1866; reprint, Lincoln: University of Nebraska Press, 1995.

Centers for Disease Control. "Smallpox Disease Overview." Accessed August 16, 2010. http://www.bt.cdc.gov/agent/smallpox/overview/disease-facts.asp.

Chambrun, Marquis de (Charles Adolphe Pineton). "Personal Recollections of Mr. Lincoln." *Scribner's* 13 (January 1893): 26–38.

Chase, Salmon P. *The Salmon P. Chase Papers.* Vol. 1, *Journals, 1829–1872.* Edited by John Niven et al. Kent, OH: Kent State University Press, 1993.

Chesson, Michael B. "An Enthusiastic Endorsement." In *The Intimate World of Abraham Lincoln*, by C. A. Tripp. New York: Free Press, 2005. 238–46.

Chicago Times, October 10, 1862.

Clark, Allan. "Abraham Lincoln in the National Capital." *Records of the Columbia Historical Society* 27 (1925): 1–174.

Clinton, Catherine. *Mrs. Lincoln: A Life.* New York: HarperCollins, 2009.

Colimore, Edward. "Lincoln's 'Shroud of Turin': City Museum Torn on DNA Request." *Philadelphia Inquirer*, April 13, 2009. www.philly.com/inquirer/local/nj/20090413_Lincoln_s_Shroud_of_Turin_.html.

Conkling Family Papers. Box, Manuscripts Department. Abraham Lincoln Presidential Library, Springfield, IL.

Craughwell, Thomas J. *Stealing Lincoln's Body*. Cambridge, MA: Belknap Press of Harvard University Press, 2007.

Crofts, Daniel W. *A Secession Crisis Enigma: William Henry Hurlbert and "The Diary of a Public Man."* Baton Rouge: Louisiana State University Press, 2010.

Davidson, Glen W. "Abraham Lincoln and the DNA Controversy." *Journal of the Abraham Lincoln Association* 17 (Winter 1996): 1–26.

David Davis Papers. Box, Manuscripts Department. Abraham Lincoln Presidential Library, Springfield, IL.

Dennett, Tyler, ed. *Lincoln and the Civil War in the Diaries and Letters of John Hay*. New York: Dodd, Mead, 1939; reprint, New York: Da Capo, 1988.

"Doctor Claims Lincoln Had Fatal Malady." *Chicago Tribune*, April 14, 1978.

Donald, David Herbert. *Lincoln*. New York: Simon and Schuster, 1995.

———. *"We Are Lincoln Men": Abraham Lincoln and His Friends*. New York: Simon and Schuster, 2003.

Durham, Harriet F. "Lincoln's Sons and the Marfan Syndrome." *Lincoln Herald* 79 (Summer 1977): 67–71.

"Edward Baker Lincoln." *Illinois State Journal* (Springfield), February 2, 1850.

Elizabeth Parker Todd Edwards Papers. SC 445, Manuscripts Department. Abraham Lincoln Presidential Library, Springfield, IL.

Ephraim Elmer Ellsworth Papers. SC 455, Manuscripts Department. Abraham Lincoln Presidential Library, Springfield, IL.

Emerson, Jason. *The Madness of Mary Lincoln*. Carbondale: Southern Illinois University Press, 2007.

———. "'Of Such Is the Kingdom of Heaven': The Mystery of 'Little Eddie.'" *Journal of the Illinois State Historical Society* 92 (Autumn 1999): 207–21.

Epstein, Daniel Mark. *The Lincolns: Portrait of a Marriage*. New York: Ballantine Books, 2008.

Evans, W. A. *Mrs. Abraham Lincoln: A Study of Her Personality and Her Influence on Lincoln*. New York: Alfred A. Knopf, 1932; reprint, Carbondale: Southern Illinois University Press, 2010.

Fessenden, Francis. *The Life and Public Services of William Pitt Fessenden*. 2 vols. New York: Houghton Mifflin, 1907.

Fishman, Ronald S., and Adriana Da Silveira. "Lincoln's Craniofacial Microsomia: Three-Dimensional Laser Scanning of Two Lincoln Life Masks." *Archives of Ophthalmology* 125 (August 2007): 1126–30.

Fleischner, Jennifer. *Mrs. Lincoln and Mrs. Keckly: The Remarkable Story of the Friendship Between a First Lady and a Former Slave.* New York: Broadway Books, 2003.

French, Benjamin Brown. *Witness to the Young Republic: A Yankee's Journal, 1828–1870.* Edited by Donald B. Cole and John J. McDonough. Hanover, NH: University Press of New England, 1989.

Furgurson, Ernest B. *Freedom Rising: Washington in the Civil War.* New York: Alfred A. Knopf, 2004.

Gannett, Lewis. "'Overwhelming Evidence' of a Lincoln–Ann Rutledge Romance? Reexamining Rutledge Family Reminiscences." *Journal of the Abraham Lincoln Association* 26 (Winter 2005): 28–41.

Garrison, Webb B. *The Lincoln No One Knows: The Mysterious Man Who Ran the Civil War.* Nashville, TN: Rutledge Hill Press, 1993.

George, Joseph, Jr. "Lincoln to Stanton: An Unpublished Letter." *Lincoln Herald* 63 (December 1961): 193–95.

Goff, John S. *Robert Todd Lincoln: A Man in His Own Right.* Norman: University of Oklahoma Press, 1968; reprint, Manchester, VT: Friends of Hildene, 1990.

Goldman, Armond S., and Frank C. Schmalstieg. "Abraham Lincoln's Gettysburg Illness." *Journal of Medical Biography* 15 (May 2007): 104–10; reprint, *Journal of Civil War Medicine* 11 (October–December 2007): 107–12.

Goodwin, Doris Kearns. *Team of Rivals: The Political Genius of Abraham Lincoln.* New York: Simon and Schuster, 2005.

Gordon, Abraham M. "Abraham Lincoln—A Medical Appraisal." *Journal of the Kentucky State Medical Association* 60 (1962): 249–53.

Grimsley, Elizabeth Todd. "Six Months in the White House." *Journal of the Illinois State Historical Society* 19 (October 1926–January 1927): 43–73.

Phineas D. Gurley Letters. SC 616, Manuscripts Department. Abraham Lincoln Presidential Library, Springfield, IL.

Hamilton, Charles, and Lloyd Ostendorf. *Lincoln in Photographs: An Album of Every Known Pose.* Norman: University of Oklahoma Press, 1963.

Hammond, William Alexander. *A Statement of the Causes Which Led to the Dismissal of Surgeon-General William A. Hammond from the Army; with a Review of the Evidence Adduced Before the Court.* New York: privately published, 1864.

Hanchett, William. "Abraham Lincoln and the Tripp Thesis." Part 4. *Lincoln Herald* 112 (Spring 2010): 7–21.

———. "Lincoln and the Tripp Thesis." Parts 1 and 2. *Lincoln Herald* 110 (Fall 2008): 158–204.

———. "Lincoln and the Tripp Thesis, Part Three." *Lincoln Herald* 111 (Summer 2009): 74–93.

———. *The Lincoln Murder Conspiracies*. Urbana: University of Illinois Press, 1983.

Harvey, Cordelia A. P. "A Wisconsin Woman's Picture of President Lincoln." *Wisconsin Magazine of History* 1 (March 1918): 233–55.

Hathaway, Jay. "Review of *The Intimate World of Abraham Lincoln*." *American Historical Review* 111 (April 2006): 483.

Helm, Katherine. *The True Story of Mary, Wife of Lincoln: Containing the Recollections of Mary Lincoln's Sister Emilie*. New York: Harper and Bros., 1928. Reprinted as *Mary, Wife of Lincoln*. Rutland, VT: W. F. Sharp, 2007.

Henry, Robert S. *The Armed Forces Institute of Pathology: Its First Century, 1862–1962*. Washington, DC: Government Printing Office, 1964.

Hirschhorn, Norbert. "Mary Lincoln's 'Suicide Attempt': A Physician Reconsiders the Evidence." *Lincoln Herald* 105 (Fall 2003): 94–98.

Hirschhorn, Norbert, and Robert G. Feldman. "Mary Lincoln's Final Illness: A Medical and Historical Reappraisal." *Journal of the History of Medicine* 54 (October 1999): 511–42.

Hirschhorn, Norbert, Robert G. Feldman, and Ian A. Greaves. "Abraham Lincoln's Blue Pills: Did Our 16th President Suffer from Mercury Poisoning?" *Perspectives in Biology and Medicine* 44 (Summer 2001): 315–32.

History of the Medical Society of the District of Columbia, 1817–1909. Washington, DC: The Society, 1909.

Holst, Erika. "'One of the Best Women I Ever Knew': Abraham Lincoln and Rebecca Pomroy." *Journal of the Abraham Lincoln Association* 31 (Summer 2010): 12–20.

Holzer, Harold, ed. *Lincoln's White House Secretary: The Adventurous Life of William O. Stoddard*. Carbondale: Southern Illinois University Press, 2007.

Hutchinson, John M. "What Was Tad Lincoln's Speech Problem?" *Journal of the Abraham Lincoln Association* 30 (Winter 2009): 35–51.

Jaquette, Henrietta Stratton, ed. *Letters of a Civil War Nurse: Cornelia Hancock, 1863–1865*. Reprint of *South after Gettysburg: Letters of Cornelia Hancock from the Army of the Potomac, 1863–1865*. Freeport, NY: Books for Libraries Press, 1971; reprint, Lincoln: University of Nebraska Press, 1998.

Johnson, Martin P. "Did Abraham Lincoln Sleep with His Bodyguard? Another Look at the Evidence." *Journal of the Abraham Lincoln Association* 27 (Summer 2006): 42–55.

Kauffman, Michael W. *American Brutus: John Wilkes Booth and the Lincoln Conspiracies*. New York: Random, 2005.

Kaye, David H. *The Double Helix and the Law of Evidence*. Cambridge, MA: Harvard University Press, 2010.

Keckley, Elizabeth. *Behind the Scenes or Thirty Years a Slave, and Four Years in the White House*. New York: G. W. Carleton, 1868; reprint, New York: Oxford University Press, 1988.

Kramer, Sidney. "Lincoln at the Fair." *Abraham Lincoln Quarterly* 3 (September 1945): 340–58.

Kunhardt, Dorothy Meserve, and Philip B. Kunhardt Jr. *Twenty Days*. New York: Castle, 1965.

Larsen, Arthur J. *Crusader and Feminist: Letters of Jane Grey Swisshelm, 1858–1865*. St. Paul: Minnesota Historical Society, 1934.

Lattimer, John K. "The Danger in Claiming that Abraham Lincoln Had the Marfan Syndrome." *Lincoln Fellowship of Wisconsin Historical Bulletin* 46 (1991): 38–47.

———. "Lincoln Did Not Have the Marfan Syndrome." *New York State Journal of Medicine* 81 (November 1981): 1805–13.

———. "The Wound That Killed Lincoln." *Journal of the American Medical Association* 187 (February 15, 1964): 480–89.

Leale, Charles A. *Lincoln's Last Hours: Address Delivered Before the Commandery of the State of New York Military Order of the Loyal Legion of the United States*. New York: privately printed, 1909.

Letters to Abraham Lincoln. SC 914-E, Manuscripts Department. Abraham Lincoln Presidential Library, Springfield, IL.

Lincoln, Abraham. *The Collected Works of Abraham Lincoln*. Edited by Roy P. Basler. 9 vols. New Brunswick, NJ: Rutgers University Press, 1953.

———. *The Collected Works of Abraham Lincoln, Supplement: 1832–1865*. Edited by Roy P. Basler. Westport, CT: Greenwood Press, 1974.

Lincoln Biohistory Study Group. Agendas and notes, in possession of Thomas F. Schwartz, member of Ethics Panel.

Lincoln Log. http://www.thelincolnlog.org.

"Lincoln's Visit to Philadelphia in June 1864." *Lincoln Lore* 1315 (June 21, 1954).

Lowry, Thomas P. *Merciful Lincoln: The President and Military Justice*. Self-published, 2009.

Lowry, Thomas P., and Jack D. Welsh. *Tarnished Scalpels: The Court-Martials of Fifty Union Surgeons*. Mechanicsburg, PA: Stackpole Books, 2000.

Marcotty, Josephine. "Mercury in Lincoln's Medicine May Have Hurt Him." *State Journal-Register* (Springfield, IL), July 18, 2001, 3.

"Marfan Syndrome." MedicineNet.com. Accessed January 12, 2011. www/medicinenet.com/marfan_syndrome.

Maxwell, William Quentin. *Lincoln's Fifth Wheel: The Political History of the United States Sanitary Commission*. New York: Longmans, Green, 1956.

Mayo Clinic. "Typhoid Fever." http://www.mayoclinic.com/health/typhoid-fever/DS00538.

McAndrew, Tara McClellan. *Stories of Springfield: Life in Lincoln's Town*. Charleston, SC: History Press, 2010.

McClintock, Russell. *Lincoln and the Decision for War: The Northern Response to Secession*. Chapel Hill: University of North Carolina Press, 2008.

McKusick, Victor A. "Advisory Statement by the Panel on DNA Testing of Abraham Lincoln's Tissue." *Caduceus* 7 (Spring 1991): 43–46.

McPherson, James M. *Tried by War: Abraham Lincoln as Commander in Chief.* New York: Penguin Press, 2008.

Micozzi, Marc S. "When the Patient Is Abraham Lincoln." *Caduceus* 7 (Spring 1991): 35–42.

Miers, Earl Schenck. *Lincoln Day by Day.* 3 vols. Washington, DC: Lincoln Sesquicentennial Commission, 1960.

Miller, Joy. "Pay Attention to Child's ADD." *Peoria Observer,* September 15, 1999.

Monroe, Dan. "Review of *The Intimate World of Abraham Lincoln* by C. A. Tripp." *Journal of Illinois History* 9 (Summer 2006): 140–41.

"Mutant Gene Shatters Nerves: Was Abe Lincoln Affected?" *Medical News Today,* January 30, 2007. www.medicalnewstoday.com/articles/61385.php.

National Archives. RG 92, Records of the Office of the Quartermaster General, 1792–1929, Correspondence, 1818–1926, Entry 225 Consolidated Correspondence File, 1794–1915, box 886 (old).

Neely, Mark E., and R. Gerald McMurtry. *The Insanity File: The Case of Mary Todd Lincoln.* Carbondale: Southern Illinois University Press, 1986.

New York Times, July 3, 1863.

Obituary. *Chicago Tribune,* July 16, 1871.

Obituary. *Illinois State Register,* July 17, 1871.

Orton, Darius. "An Eyewitness Account." *Lincoln Herald* 77 (Spring 1975): 68.

"The Parent and the Politician." *Chicago Press and Tribune,* June 29, 1860.

Pearson, Emmet F. "Abraham Lincoln—Health, Habits and Doctors." *Illinois Medical Journal* 147 (February 1975): 143–47, 174.

———. "Tragic Deaths of the Lincoln Sons." *Illinois Medical Journal* (November 1968); reprinted in *itam: Magazine about Tuberculosis and Respiratory Disease* 32 (February 1970): 230–34.

Pinsker, Matthew. "Review of *The Intimate World of Abraham Lincoln.*" *Journal of American History* 92 (March 2006): 1442–43.

Porter, Horace. *Campaigning with Grant.* New York: Century Co., 1897; reprint, Alexandria, VA: Time-Life, 1981.

Pratt, Harry E. *The Personal Finances of Abraham Lincoln.* Springfield, IL: Abraham Lincoln Association, 1943.

Prokopowicz, Gerald J. *Did Lincoln Own Slaves? And Other Frequently Asked Questions about Abraham Lincoln.* New York: Pantheon, 2008.

Rafuse, Ethan S. "Typhoid and Tumult: Lincoln's Response to General McClellan's Bout with Typhoid Fever during the Winter of 1861–62." *Journal of the Abraham Lincoln Association* 18 (Summer 1997): 1–16.

Randall, Ruth Painter. *Lincoln's Sons.* Boston: Little, Brown, 1955.

Read, Harry. "A Hand to Hold While Dying: Dr. Charles A. Leale at Lincoln's Side." *Lincoln Herald* 79 (Spring 1977): 21–26.

Reilly, Philip R. *Abraham Lincoln's DNA and Other Adventures in Genetics.* Cold Spring Harbor, NY: Cold Spring Harbor Laboratory Press, 2000.

"Research Hints at an Ailment in Lincoln." *New York Times*, January 28, 2006, A18.

Moses P. Rice et al. to Lincoln, ca. March 3, 1863. Lincoln Collection. Abraham Lincoln Presidential Library, Springfield, IL.

Robbins, Jefferson. "Writer Asserts Proof Lincoln Was Gay." *State Journal-Register* (Springfield, IL), May 16, 1999, 1.

Robinson, Tara Rodden. *Genetics for Dummies*. 2nd ed. Hoboken, NJ: Wiley, 2010.

Ross, Rodney A. "Mary Todd Lincoln, Patient at Bellevue Place, Batavia." *Journal of the Illinois State Historical Society* 63 (Spring 1970): 5–34.

Schroeder-Lein, Glenna R. *The Encyclopedia of Civil War Medicine*. Armonk, NY: M. E. Sharpe, 2008.

———. "Lincoln and the Great Central Sanitary Fair." *Lincoln Editor* 2 (July–September 2002): 1–2.

Schroeder-Lein, Glenna R., and Richard Zuczek. *Andrew Johnson: A Biographical Companion*. Santa Barbara, CA: ABC-Clio, 2001.

Schwartz, Barry. "Ann Rutledge in American Memory: Social Change and the Erosion of a Romantic Drama." *Journal of the Abraham Lincoln Association* 26 (Winter 2005): 1–27.

Schwartz, Harold. "Abraham Lincoln and Cardiac Decompensation: A Preliminary Report." *Western Journal of Medicine* 128 (February 1978): 174–77.

———. "Abraham Lincoln and the Marfan Syndrome." *Journal of the American Medical Association* 187 (February 15, 1964): 473–79.

Schwartz, Thomas F. "'My stay on Earth is growing very short': Mary Todd Lincoln's Letters to Willis Danforth and Elizabeth Swing." *Journal of Illinois History* 6 (Summer 2003): 125–36.

———. "Whither *The Collected Works of Abraham Lincoln*? More Unpublished Lincoln Letters." *Journal of the Abraham Lincoln Association* 13 (1992): 47–56.

Schwartz, Thomas F., and Kim Bauer. "Unpublished Mary Todd Lincoln." *Journal of the Abraham Lincoln Association* 17 (Summer 1996): 1–21.

Searcher, Victor. *Lincoln's Journey to Greatness: A Factual Account of the Twelve-Day Inaugural Trip*. Philadelphia: John C. Winston, 1960.

Shenk, Joshua Wolf. *Lincoln's Melancholy: How Depression Challenged a President and Fueled His Greatness*. Boston: Houghton Mifflin, 2005.

Shutes, Milton H. *Lincoln and the Doctors: A Medical Narrative of the Life of Abraham Lincoln*. New York: Pioneer Press, 1933.

———. "Mortality of the Five Lincoln Boys." *Lincoln Herald* 57 (Spring 1955): 3–11.

Simon, John Y. "Abraham Lincoln and Ann Rutledge." *Journal of the Abraham Lincoln Association* 11 (1990): 13–33.

Smith, Adam I. P. "Lincoln Scholarship and the Return of Intimacy." *Journal of the Abraham Lincoln Association* 27 (Summer 2006): 56–71.

Sotos, John G. *The Physical Lincoln Complete 1.1a*. Mt. Vernon, VA: Mt. Vernon Book Systems, 2008.

Speed, Joshua F. "Incidents in the Early Life of A. Lincoln." SC 1443-A, Manuscripts Department. Abraham Lincoln Presidential Library, Springfield, IL.

Spiegel, Allen D. *A. Lincoln, Esquire: A Shrewd, Sophisticated Lawyer in His Time*. Macon, GA: Mercer University Press, 2002.

Steers, Edward, Jr. *Blood on the Moon: The Assassination of Abraham Lincoln*. Lexington: University Press of Kentucky, 2001.

———. *Lincoln Legends, Myths, Hoaxes, and Confabulations Associated with Our Greatest President*. Lexington: University Press of Kentucky, 2007.

Stillé, Charles J. *Memorial of the Great Central Fair for the U.S. Sanitary Commission*. Philadelphia: U.S. Sanitary Commission, 1864.

Stoddard, William O. *Inside the White House in War Times: Memoirs and Reports of Lincoln's Secretary*. Edited by Michael Burlingame. Lincoln: University of Nebraska Press, 2000.

Strong, George Templeton. *Diary of the Civil War, 1860–1865*. Edited by Allan Nevins. New York: Macmillan, 1962.

"Study Traces Gene Defect in Abe's Family." *State Journal-Register* (Springfield, IL), November 2, 1994, 10.

Symonds, Craig L. *Lincoln and His Admirals: Abraham Lincoln, the U.S. Navy, and the Civil War*. New York: Oxford University Press, 2008.

Taft, Charles Sabin. *Abraham Lincoln's Last Hours*. Chicago: Black Cat Press, 1968.

———. "Notes of the circumstances attending the assassination of Abraham Lincoln . . ." Joseph N. Nathanson Collection of Lincolniana. Accessed September 21, 2010. http://digital.library.mcgill.ca/lincoln/images/exhibit/4/big/Taft%20Journal%2001.jpg.

Taylor Family (James M.) Papers. Box, Manuscripts Department. Abraham Lincoln Presidential Library, Springfield, IL.

Temple, Wayne C. "A. W. French: Lincoln Family Dentist." *Lincoln Herald* 63 (Fall 1961): 151–54.

———. *Dr. Anson G. Henry: Personal Physician to the Lincolns*. Bulletin of the 44th Annual Meeting of the Lincoln Fellowship of Wisconsin, Milwaukee, 1987.

———. "Lincoln in the Census." *Lincoln Herald* 68 (Fall 1966): 135–40.

Todt, Ron. "Test of Lincoln's DNA Sought to Prove Cancer Theory." *State Journal-Register* (Springfield, IL), April 18, 2009.

"Tombstone of Lincoln's Second Son, Lost for 89 Years, Found in Oak Ridge." *Illinois State Register* (Springfield), September 8, 1954.

Trefousse, Hans Louis. "Belated Revelations of the Assassination Committee." *Lincoln Herald* 58 (Spring–Summer 1956): 13–16.

Tripp, C. A. *The Intimate World of Abraham Lincoln*. New York: Free Press, 2005.

Turner, Justin G., and Linda Levitt Turner. *Mary Todd Lincoln: Her Life and Letters*. New York: Knopf, 1972.

Turner, Thomas R. "Editor's Introduction." *Lincoln Herald* 110 (Fall 2008): 156–57.

US Census. Mortality Schedule, 1850, Illinois, Sangamon, Springfield, 787. Accessed at ancestry.com.

US Census. 1860, Washington, DC, Ward 3, 30. Accessed at ancestry.com.

Washington Evening Star, August 29, 1862.

Welles, Gideon. *Diary of Gideon Welles*. 3 vols. Edited by Howard K. Beale. 1911; reprint, New York: W. W. Norton, 1960.

White, Ronald C., Jr. *A. Lincoln: A Biography*. New York: Random House, 2009.

———. *The Eloquent President: A Portrait of Lincoln through His Words*. New York: Random House, 2005.

Whitney, Henry Clay. *Life on the Circuit with Lincoln*. Boston: Estes and Lauriat, 1892.

Who Was Who in America: Historical Volume, 1607–1896. Chicago: Marquis, 1963.

"Why Abe Was No Beauty." *Atlanta Journal and Constitution*, February 9, 1975, 20-C.

Wilson, Douglas L. *Honor's Voice*. New York: Alfred A. Knopf, 1998.

Wilson, Douglas L., and Rodney O. Davis. *Herndon's Informants: Letters, Interviews, and Statements about Abraham Lincoln*. Urbana: University of Illinois Press, 1998.

Worthington, Daniel E. "The Open Polar Sea: Abraham Lincoln and an Arctic Explorer." *Lincoln Editor* 10 (July–September 2010): 6–7.

INDEX

Kidwell, Dr., 63
Kincaid, Robert, 50
King, Albert F. A., 76
Kinsey, Alfred, 50–52, 55
Kramer, Larry, 50

Lamb, Brian, 50
Lamon, Ward Hill, 14, 16
Lattimer, John K., 40
laudanum, 85
Lawson, Thomas, 56
Leale, Charles A., 74–79
Leech, Margaret, 50
lens dislocation, 39
Lincoln (Donald), xii
Lincoln, Abraham: and accidents,
1–2, 6; and Ann Rutledge, 3; and
aortic insufficiency, 38, 40; and
apples, 16; assassination of, 74–
79; asymmetrical head of, 41; and
ataxia, xi, 45; attacked by blacks,
2; autopsy of, 46–47, 77–78; and
ax, 6, 35; and bad weather, 3–4;
battlefield visits of, 34; body of,
attempt to steal, 46; breakdown
of, 3–5; and broken engagement,
4; and cancer, 41, 44; and cardiovascular problems, 37–38, 40;
childhood of, 1–2; cold hands
and feet of, 32, 40–41; and colds,
17; and congestive heart failure,
37–38, 40; and constipation, 5, 14,
40–41; and courts-martial, 62–63;
as crazy, 3–5; and daily carriage
rides, 18; death of, 68, 77, 80, 83;
and depression, 2–8, 26, 28, 32, 40;
descriptions of, 17–18, 26–27, 30–
31, 33–35, 51; diet of, 3, 18, 25; and
DNA testing, 45–49; drowning of
averted, 1; embalming of, 79; and
epilepsy, 2; and exercise, 16, 35, 39;
and exhaustion, 4, 17–18, 26–27,
32–35; and eyeglasses, 16, 39; and
eye problems, 2, 16, 39; faints, 18,
32, 41, 43; far-sightedness of, 16,
39; feet of, 5, 26, 32, 39–41, 63; flat-

footed gait of, 15, 41, 45; funeral
journey of, 79; and Gettysburg
trip, 28–29; good health of noted,
30–32, 35; and headaches, 2, 12,
14, 16, 18, 25, 29, 35–36, 41; head
wound of, 74–79; and homosexuality, xi, 37, 49–55; and hospital
chaplains, 61; and hospital visits,
35, 64–66; and humor, 6, 30; and
hypochondriasis, 5, 14; illness (unspecified) of, 6, 8, 25–27, 31–36; injuries to, 2, 6, 8, 26; and insomnia,
15, 18, 26; kicked in head by horse,
2; last hours of, 74–77; as lawyer,
3, 13, 56; life casts of, 39, 41; and
lip bumps, 41, 44; and low muscle
tone, 6, 41; and malaria, 2–3, 5, 8,
19, 22; and Marfan syndrome, xi,
37–40, 45–48, 77, 82, 88; marriage
of, 5, 8–9, 53, 55; and melancholy
temperament, 5–6; and MEN2B,
xi, 6, 40–41, 44–45, 48–49, 83;
and mercury poisoning, xi, 15–16;
and nerve damage, 2; office hours
of, 18; and overwork, 17–18; and
patronage, 17, 60–62, 64; and
pensions, 67; and photographs,
35, 41, 44; photographs of, 42–43;
physical decline of, 35–36, 40–41,
44, 78; and plays, 29, 74; and poetry, 6, 25; poisoning of attempted,
32–33; political campaigning by, 4;
as presidential candidate, 12; privacy of, 47, 49; and puberty, 50–51;
and reading, 18, 25; and Reconstruction, 33; and relaxation, 18,
27, 31, 33–35, 74; sadness of, 5–6,
26–27; and sanitary fairs, 68–72;
and seasickness, 26, 31, 34; and secession crisis, 17; and Shakespeare,
6; and smallpox, 29–30, 44; and
soldier health needs, 66–67; and
sore throat, 12; speeches by, 17,
70–71; and sprained wrist, 26;
as state legislator, 4–6; strength
of, 35–36, 39–40, 78; and stress,

Glenna R. Schroeder-Lein is manuscripts librarian for the non-Lincoln manuscripts at the Abraham Lincoln Presidential Library in Springfield, Illinois. Her previous publications include *The Encyclopedia of Civil War Medicine*, *Confederate Hospitals on the Move: Samuel H. Stout and the Army of Tennessee*, and *Andrew Johnson: A Biographical Companion* (with Richard Zuczek).

CONCISE
LINCOLN
LIBRARY

This series of concise books fills a need for short studies of the life, times, and legacy of President Abraham Lincoln. Each book gives readers the opportunity to quickly achieve basic knowledge of a Lincoln-related topic. These books bring fresh perspectives to well-known topics, investigate previously overlooked subjects, and explore in greater depth topics that have not yet received book-length treatment. For a complete list of current and forthcoming titles, see www.conciselincolnlibrary.com.

Other Books in the Concise Lincoln Library

Abraham Lincoln and Horace Greeley
Gregory A. Borchard

Lincoln and the Civil War
Michael Burlingame

Lincoln and the Constitution
Brian R. Dirck

Lincoln and the Election of 1860
Michael S. Green

Lincoln and Race
Richard Striner

Lincoln as Hero
Frank J. Williams

Abraham and Mary Lincoln
Kenneth J. Winkle